T.

Spiritual Care for
Healthcare Professionals

Spiritual Care for Healthcare Professionals

Reflecting on clinical practice

TOM GORDON
Chair
Chaplaincy Training Advisory Group, Scotland

EWAN KELLY
Programme Director
Spiritual Care and Healthcare Chaplaincy, NHS Education for Scotland
Senior Lecturer in Pastoral Theology, University of Edinburgh

and

DAVID MITCHELL
Programme Leader, Healthcare Chaplaincy
Lecturer in Palliative Care
University of Glasgow

Foreword by

STEPHEN THORNTON CBE
Chief Executive
The Health Foundation

Radcliffe Publishing
London • New York

Radcliffe Publishing Ltd
33–41 Dallington Street
London
EC1V 0BB
United Kingdom

www.radcliffepublishing.com

Electronic catalogue and worldwide online ordering facility.

British Library Cataloguing in Publication Data

A catalogue record for this book is available from the British Library.

ISBN-13: 978 184619 455 9

The paper used for the text pages of this book
is FSC® certified. FSC (The Forest Stewardship
Council®) is an international network to promote
responsible management of the world's forests.

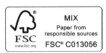

Typeset by Phoenix Photosetting, Chatham, Kent
Printed and bound by TJI Digital, Padstow, Cornwall

Contents

Foreword

Here is a book that fills a gap for all those seeking to understand the spiritual components of healthcare and how to meet them. Written for all healthcare professionals, including chaplains and spiritual care workers, it offers insights and practical advice aplenty.

This book does not pull its punches. 'The core skills of a healthcare chaplain,' the authors write, 'include enabling others to articulate their sense of spirituality, acting as a resource for staff and volunteers in their assessment and delivery of spiritual care. Encouraging healthcare professionals to develop their self-awareness and competence with regard to spirituality and spiritual care is an essential capability and competence for the chaplain.' Just reading Chapter 1 will be a real challenge for many.

It is said that times are tough for healthcare chaplains in the NHS today. I think it was ever thus. As a young trainee administrator in the early 1980s, I recall checking admission forms from the night before in an unnamed teaching hospital somewhere in the north of England. As was so often the case, the section marked 'religion' had been left blank, so I was instructed to write in 'C of E'. No shared decision making there, then! Indeed, there has never been a golden age where the spiritual preferences and desires of patients, carers and staff were taken seriously and given their due place. It was and will always be counter-cultural to some extent.

What this book does is to provide practical help to those with a responsibility to lead in this field. It starts powerfully by stating that the greatest difficulty is overcoming the confusion between spiritual care and religion. 'Many people when saying the word "spiritual" are actually thinking "religion",' say the authors. 'Indeed, not that long ago a spiritual assessment on admission to a hospital ward was a single question: "What religion are you?" Although religion may feature in a person's spirituality, it will be alongside a host of other aspects, such as family, friends, work, health, love and leisure activities.'

The book then goes on to offer practical help and advice for occasions when one would expect the spiritual components of care to be at their most intense: loss, grief, bereavement, staff support, etc. And it does so by asking the reader, chapter by chapter, to undertake a 'reflective activity', a technique that I am sure has wider utility in all aspects of healthcare management and decision making.

But what marks out this book for me is Chapter 11: Nurturing our spiritual selves. 'How,' ask the authors, 'do we as healthcare professionals... process our experiences of supporting distressed service users and the emotions, issues and questions that are raised in us? Where is the balm in our lives to soothe and care for our souls? How may we learn and grow in an understanding of ourselves and our practice, as individuals and as teams working in relationship, from reflecting on experience?' So, if you want my advice, this is the place to start.

Stephen Thornton CBE
Chief Executive, The Health Foundation
Non Executive Director, Monitor
Expert Member, Department of Health National Quality Board
June 2011

About the authors

Tom Gordon is a Church of Scotland minister who for 15 years was a hospice chaplain with Marie Curie Cancer Care (MCCC) in their Edinburgh hospice and acted as adviser to MCCC in spiritual and religious care. He also served for several years as President of the Association of Hospice and Palliative Care Chaplains, and is currently chair of the Chaplaincy Training Advisory Group in Scotland. He now devotes his time to writing and lecturing, as well as facilitating the Acorns Bereavement Support Programmes in Edinburgh and the Lothians.

Ewan Kelly is a former junior doctor who has spent most of his working life as a healthcare chaplain and a university teacher. His experience includes chaplaincy both in two teaching hospitals and in an independent hospice. He currently works with NHS Education for Scotland on the strategic development of spiritual care and healthcare chaplaincy in NHS Scotland as Programme Director for Chaplaincy and Spiritual Care. In addition, he has a part-time position as Senior Lecturer in Pastoral Theology at the University of Edinburgh.

David Mitchell is the programme leader for healthcare chaplaincy and university teacher in palliative care at the University of Glasgow. He is also a parish minister in West Cowal, Argyll, distance learning tutor for Edith Cowan University, Western Australia, and executive member of the UK Board of Healthcare Chaplaincy. His previous experience includes time as a chaplain and lecturer in palliative care with Marie Curie Cancer Care, as a consultant in healthcare chaplaincy for NHS Education for Scotland, and as joint editor of the *Scottish Journal of Healthcare Chaplaincy*.

Acknowledgements

The authors gratefully acknowledge the support and affirmation of many colleagues who have been or are currently involved in healthcare chaplaincy throughout the UK, as well as professional colleagues from many other healthcare disciplines. These individuals have, specifically and unknowingly, been a great asset during the conceptualisation and preparation of this book. In particular, many thanks are due to Georgina Nelson and Mark Stobert for generously giving their time and insight when reviewing the manuscript at draft stage, to Gillian Nineham and Jamie Etherington at Radcliffe Publishing for their unfailing encouragement and guidance, and to Stephen Thornton for his willingness to write the Foreword and for the generosity of spirit contained in his words.

We are also grateful to SPCK and Bloodaxe Books for permission to reproduce the poems by Kathy Galloway and Stewart Conn.

Introduction

Professional healthcare organisations and health departments regularly include statements in their codes of conduct, professional guidelines, standards and capability and competency frameworks that spiritual care is an integral part of the practitioner's professional role.[1-5]

The guidance for NHS staff in the publication *Spiritual Care Matters* states:

> Spiritual care in the NHS must be both inclusive and accepting of human difference. As we learn to listen better to the particular needs of different people, so we equip ourselves for work that is more fulfilling and effective. The provision of spiritual care by NHS staff is not yet another demand on their hard pressed time. It is the essence of their work and it enables and promotes healing in the fullest sense to all parties, both giver and receiver, of such care.[6]

This book has been written to tease out what these numerous statements, guidelines and standards mean, and to equip healthcare professionals with the knowledge, skills and competence to provide this 'essence' of spiritual care within their professional practice. The book also aims to guide the reader in exploring how spiritual care is fundamentally relational in nature and inherent in the professional art of providing healthcare.

The authors expect this book to encourage healthcare professionals to be open to the enormous breadth and diversity in individual spirituality, and how this can enhance and develop healthcare practice. However, there are a number of overarching questions on which the authors have a clear response. For example, who provides spiritual care? What is the relationship between spirituality and religion? What is the relationship between spirituality and humanism or atheism?

WHO PROVIDES SPIRITUAL CARE?

The authors share the view expressed above, and consider that all healthcare professionals have the potential to provide spiritual care and can do so as part of their regular practice. However, as with all aspects of healthcare, spiritual care can have a complexity that will require specialist knowledge, expertise and experience to assess and meet the needs of patients and their carers, and this expertise is provided by a healthcare chaplain or a specialist spiritual care provider.

SPIRITUALITY AND RELIGION

The greatest difficulty in spiritual care is overcoming the confusion with religion. Many people when saying the word 'spiritual' are actually thinking 'religion.' Indeed, not that long ago a spiritual assessment on admission to a hospital ward consisted of a single question: 'What religion are you?' Although religion may feature in a person's spirituality, it will be alongside a host of other aspects, such as family, friends, work, health, love and leisure activities.

The authors firmly believe that the only way to understand spirituality and its relationship to religion is to start within ourselves. The first chapters in this book aim to do just that. The reader is encouraged to work through a process of self-awareness and then to integrate their experiences of faith, belief and culture to form an understanding of their spirituality, and to appreciate the diversity of spirituality. In Chapter 6, the complexities of the relationship between spirituality and religion are explored by 'disentangling spiritual and religious care'.

SPIRITUALITY AND HUMANISM

Another common misconception is that spirituality is irrelevant to those who adopt a secular, atheist or humanist perspective on life and living. All people, regardless of their life stance, have an innate spirituality. Indeed most of the recent developments in standards, guidelines and competences in spiritual and religious care have been informed and embraced by representatives of the humanist societies. There are also humanists employed and serving in NHS chaplaincy services providing spiritual care. The authors' view is that spirituality is individual to each person and can include all religious faiths, belief groups (such as humanists), and those of any life stance.

WHO IS THIS BOOK FOR?

First and foremost, this book is a practical guide for healthcare professionals of all disciplines. It encourages the reader to reflect on their personal and professional experiences and perceptions of life, health, illness, dying and death. It guides the reader through the core skills of spiritual care, and promotes recognition of their natural abilities and instincts. Both through experience and through the use of case scenarios and reflective activities this book seeks to earth spiritual care in day-to-day professional practice.

The book has also been prepared as a core textbook and resource for further education and higher education institutions. The content has its roots in spiritual and religious care capability and competency frameworks that are recognised by the UK Departments of Health, NHS education specialists and healthcare chaplaincy organisations. As such it is a valuable resource for developing course materials and integrating spiritual care within new and existing healthcare programmes at all levels. The book is structured to aid reflective practice and to facilitate the development of self-awareness. It is not so much a traditional textbook as an instructional guidebook. The underlying premise of the book is the authors' belief that a healthcare practitioner's humanity, the self, is the most effective therapeutic tool that they possess.

The book is also a resource for healthcare chaplains. At the end of each chapter there is a section devoted to the complexity of the topic and the specialist knowledge, skills and abilities required of the chaplain or spiritual care lead.

USING THIS BOOK

The first chapters in this book lead us to explore the art of spiritual care by encouraging us to focus on our self-awareness of the core elements of spiritual care:

➤ how we understand spirituality (Chapter 1)
➤ how faith, belief and culture influence our spirituality (Chapter 2)
➤ how we can develop and use communication skills in spiritual care (Chapter 3)
➤ how teamwork can support spiritual care (Chapter 4)
➤ how we can recognise and develop competence in spiritual care (Chapter 5).

Through each of these chapters we first look at ourselves and explore what we think about spirituality, religion, life, health, illness, dying and death. From this self-awareness we then move out to consider how our own understanding of spirituality can support us in our personal and professional knowledge, skills and actions. The process of self-awareness is then used to guide us to consider how we might provide quality and informed spiritual care as part of our everyday professional practice.

From this initial understanding of spiritual care the book then goes on to add depth to spiritual care practice by encouraging the reader to consider the core elements of spiritual care in more detail, and it adds increasing complexity to enable healthcare professionals to appraise and develop their personal and professional practice. This is approached through chapters that explore the more complex aspects of providing spiritual care, namely:

➤ disentangling spiritual and religious care (Chapter 6)
➤ spiritual assessment (Chapter 7)
➤ responding to spiritual and religious needs (Chapter 8).

The complexity increases as we consider two areas where our self-awareness and clinical experience are important factors that influence the following:

➤ ethics and spiritual care (Chapter 9)

➤ the impact of loss, grief and bereavement in spiritual care (Chapter 10).

Following this in-depth analysis of spiritual care practice, the reader is then encouraged to consider how the work of spiritual care affects them personally, to engage in reflection and to consider the implications and resources of providing spiritual care in a healthcare setting. This is achieved through two chapters which address the following:

➤ processing our own spiritual journey (Chapter 11)

➤ the institution and staff support (Chapter 12).

The final chapter of the book reflects on the unique role of the chaplain in spiritual care in a healthcare setting – as chaplain to the institution (Chapter 13). The role demands the creative gift of recognising significant events in the life of the institution and an ability to assess the spiritual needs of the institution. It also involves an ability to develop trusted relationships with healthcare staff across the institution and to work with others to mark or pastorally care for all those affected by these events with confidence and understanding.

REFERENCES

1 Welsh Assembly Government. *Standards for Spiritual Care Services in the NHS in Wales in 2010*. Cardiff: Welsh Assembly Government; 2010.

2 UK Board of Healthcare Chaplaincy. *Standards for NHS Chaplaincy Services*. Cambridge: UK Board of Healthcare Chaplaincy; 2009.

3 Nursing and Midwifery Council. *Code of Conduct*. London: Nursing and Midwifery Council; 2008.

4 NHS Education for Scotland. *Spiritual Care Matters: an introductory resource for all NHS Scotland staff*. Edinburgh: NHS Education for Scotland; 2009.

5 National Institute for Clinical Excellence. *Improving Supportive and Palliative Care for Adults with Cancer. Manual*. London: National Institute for Clinical Excellence; 2004.

6 NHS Education for Scotland. *Spiritual Care Matters: an introductory resource for all NHS Scotland staff*, op. cit.

CHAPTER 1

Self-awareness

INTRODUCTION

Definitions of spirituality often include words which, although recognisable, are difficult to pin down and open to a wide variety of interpretations – for example, a sense of meaning, purpose, value, being, relationship or transcendence. This chapter will seek to grasp this ethereal term 'spirituality' and ground it in such a way that healthcare professionals can understand it and use it to inform the provision of spiritual care for patients, family/carers, volunteers and colleagues.

UNDERSTANDING SPIRITUALITY

The search for an inclusive definition of the term 'spirituality' is an elusive one. In practice, when writing on spirituality authors begin with their own definition of spirituality and develop their thinking from there. Traditional healthcare models suggest that a definition would be a good starting place. If, as a healthcare professional, you know what spirituality is, you can then develop a strategy to assess the spiritual needs of the individual and seek to address them. However, the authors take a different approach and believe that the search for a working definition of spirituality is a futile one. Spirituality is about people, and every person is different. The key to providing spiritual care is to understand what spirituality means to the person you are caring for.

Understanding spirituality is further complicated by the common misconception that spiritual care and religious care are one and the same thing. Many healthcare professionals *say* the word 'spiritual', but in their head are *thinking* 'religion'. The secular agenda, on the other hand, tries to remove religion from spirituality. The authors believe that neither of these approaches is helpful. Religion may or may not be a part of a person's spirituality, and the only way to find out is to engage with the individual. The disentangling of spirituality and religion is explored in detail in Chapter 6. In the present chapter the authors will prepare the reader by exploring and developing an inclusive understanding of spirituality.

To understand spirituality in a healthcare context and in practice it is necessary to begin with a process of self-awareness and ask the following questions.

➤ What does spirituality mean for me?
➤ What do I think and believe about the key issues of life, health, illness, dying and death?

Reflective Activity 1.1 will help you to tease out these questions and think through how you understand and interpret your spirituality.

Reflective Activity 1.1

What does spirituality mean for you or what makes life worth living?

One way to think about this is to ask yourself what gives you meaning or a sense of purpose in life (or what is most important to you in life). Try to think of four elements and place them in order of importance or significance for you:

1

2

3

4

To this list you can now add how or where you find inspiration, hope, joy and support to cope with life and living:

1

2

3

4

Does this reflect your sense of spirituality? If not, try to think what is missing.

Although there will inevitably be variations in the reader's response to this activity, in the authors' experience there are some common expressions that are prevalent on a human level, and in particular for healthcare professionals. When considering what gives you a sense of meaning and purpose, your answers might include family, friends, work, health, religion or faith. Although family and friends are consistently at the top of this list, healthcare professionals often rate work highly, and it features as an important part of their spirituality and who they are as a person. This is not surprising – if we value human relationships highly as part of who we are, then the caring professions bring us face to face with humanity when it is particularly vulnerable, and the desire to help others feeds our sense of meaning, purpose and relationship.

When we think more widely about how or where we find inspiration, hope, support and coping strategies, the list is much longer and more varied, and can include walking, music, gardening, socialising, sport, art, religion and faith, and meditation, for example. It is when we move beyond our sense of meaning and purpose to consider what sustains and inspires us in spirit that we truly enter the domain of how individual spirituality really is. Some may find their support in solitude and doing something different, others find that immersing themselves with healthy people is a good way to cope, while yet others may use both, depending on where they are and how they are feeling. There is no right or wrong way in spirituality. Rather it is a continuing journey of experience and development as well as re-connecting with previously utilised coping mechanisms which were found to be helpful.

UNDERSTANDING LIFE, HEALTH, ILLNESS, DYING AND DEATH

If spirituality is an individual and fluid concept that we journey through, then it follows that our lived experience will have an influence on our sense of spirituality, and our life experiences will have the potential to colour our understanding. Healthcare professionals often find themselves working at the challenging interface between the human experience and its transitions through life, health, illness, dying and death.

To engage with and understand spirituality, it is also important for individuals to reflect on their own perceptions and attitudes to the challenges and vulnerabilities in life, living and dying. For example, when does life begin? What does it mean to say that you are healthy? What is quality of life? What is a good death?

Reflective Activity 1.2 will help you to explore what you think and believe about some of the key issues of life, health, illness, dying and death.

Reflective Activity 1.2

This activity will use your experiences both as a person and as a healthcare professional to help you to consider your beliefs about life, health, illness, dying and death.

Health
Try writing a short statement about what 'being healthy' means to you. Consider the physical, psychological, social and spiritual factors that influence your thinking.

Illness
Reflect on an illness that you have experienced, no matter how minor.
• What was the impact of your experience on your understanding of 'being healthy'?
• From your experiences as a healthcare professional, are there any particular illnesses that you fear for yourself? Can you articulate what it is that you fear?

Life and death
While we have no say in how we come into life, we can think about how it might end.
• Think about what kind of death you envisage as a good death for yourself. For example, would it be sudden or with time to say goodbye? Would you die in your sleep or fighting to the last?

(continued)

- If you died in any of these ways, what might be the effect on your loved ones?
- Have your views changed over time? If so, what influenced this change?

Having reflected on your awareness of life, health, illness, dying and death, you can revisit Reflective Activity 1.1 and consider whether there are any additions or changes that you would like to make with regard to what spirituality means to you.

SEXUALITY AND SEXUAL PRACTICE

Why include a section on sexuality alongside self-awareness in spiritual care? The link between spirituality and sexuality is a direct rather than tenuous one. If we consider that human relationships are important factors in our sense of spirituality and who we are as a person (*see* Reflective Activity 1.1), then it follows that anything which affects those relationships affects our spirituality. Illness, treatments and drugs can all affect our sense of self, our body image and our relationships. In a very real sense the physical, psychological, social and spiritual dimensions of our being come together in our sexuality and our sense and expression of self.

In the authors' experience, the same wariness and fears that healthcare professionals have about approaching spiritual care exist around sexuality and sexual practice. For example, it is the patient's private life, the issues can be embarrassing to talk about, and there is a perceived potential for causing offence. These are legitimate fears. However, they can be overcome with self-awareness, practice and developing experience.

As with spiritual care, a useful way of approaching this issue is to explore our self-awareness – to reflect on our own thoughts and feelings about the issues of sexuality and sexual practice. From this base as healthcare professionals we may become more confident and willing to engage with patients and their family/carers.

The activities in this section will guide us in reflecting on our intimate relationships, how they might be affected by illness, and the implications that this may have for our sexuality.

Reflective Activity 1.3

Reflect on a significant relationship in your life in which your sexuality is a significant factor.

Think through the different components of the relationship and how important they are to you – for example, body image, emotions, physical contact.

After being diagnosed with an illness that you are unfamiliar with, you are being advised to undertake a course of treatment which you are told may have 'significant side-effects'. How would you respond to a healthcare professional asking you the following question?

'When given this diagnosis, patients often have concerns or questions about their sexuality. Is there anything you would like to ask?'
- Would you want to engage in the conversation to find out more?
- Would you simply answer 'no' and close the conversation?

There is no right or wrong answer to Reflective Activity 1.3. It is your choice that matters. However, if the healthcare professional does not ask the question you won't have the choice. Reflective Activity 1.4 will help you to take your thinking further and challenge the depth of your awareness and experiences.

Reflective Activity 1.4

This activity will help you to explore what information you would want to know if you were a patient about to undergo treatment that could affect your sexuality or sexual practice.

Tick the relevant boxes if you would want to know the information if you might experience any of the following:

☐ Loss of libido

☐ Dryness or pain during sex

☐ Incontinence

☐ Infertility

☐ Impotence

Are there any other areas you would add to this list?

You can also consider the following:
- Would you still want to know this information if the effects were likely to be temporary rather than permanent?
- Would your views change depending on whether or not you were in a relationship? Would you want your spouse or partner to be included in the information giving?
- Would your views have been the same if you were younger or older than you are now?

As an example of how self-awareness can influence thinking and practice, Reflective Activity 1.5 will encourage you to take your awareness of your own thinking and needs and use this to consider your workplace practices and procedures.

Reflective Activity 1.5

This activity will help you to consider your workplace setting and the implications of the care that you offer to patients and their spouses/partners for their sexuality or sexual practice.

List the treatments, drugs or elements of care that you normally provide to patients that could have an impact on their sexuality or sexual practice.

1

2

3

4

Consider the following questions:
- Is there a local protocol in place with regard to who informs the patient of the risks and/or side-effects?
- Is the information given to everyone, or are some individuals excluded because of their age or any other factor?
- Is this something that you feel your department does well?
- Are there ways in which it could be improved?

In considering our own sense of spirituality, our sense of sexuality and our understanding of life, health, dying and death, we have hopefully gained some self-awareness of where we are and what we understand about ourselves. From this base we are now better prepared to study spiritual care in depth and to journey with others. The remaining chapters of this book will guide us through that process, adding depth to our understanding of spiritual care and helping us to think through the knowledge skills and experiences that are needed to practise and provide spiritual care.

CHAPLAIN OR SPIRITUAL CARE PROFESSIONAL

As a chaplain or spiritual care professional we are expected to have an advanced self-awareness of our own spirituality, and an understanding of the broad and individual range of expressions of spirituality that are possible and unique to each person. Although we are not expected to have the answer to practical questions about sexuality and treatment side-effects, we do need an understanding of the depth and importance of these issues to individuals if we are to provide spiritual care in complex pastoral encounters. This understanding should also extend to those whom we would refer on when these questions arise.

The core skills of a healthcare chaplain include enabling others to articulate their sense of spirituality, and acting as a resource for staff and volunteers in their assessment and delivery of spiritual care. Encouraging healthcare professionals to develop their self-awareness and competence with regard to spirituality and spiritual care is an essential capability and competence for the chaplain.[1,2]

Reflective Activity 1.6 will help you to consider practical ways in which you can encourage and support healthcare professionals in their spiritual understanding and self-awareness.

Reflective Activity 1.6

You have been asked to present a teaching session on spirituality and spiritual care for healthcare professionals in training (or an induction session for new staff). From your experience of the healthcare literature on spirituality and spiritual care, and reflection on your own spirituality and practice of spiritual care:

- Identify the key concepts of spirituality.
- Prepare your introduction for the session.
- Develop an activity that would encourage those whom you are teaching to reflect on what spirituality is to them and begin the process of self-awareness.

One approach to this activity would be to take the key concepts of spirituality that you identified in Reflective Activity 1.6 and create your own understanding and working definition of spirituality. However, an alternative would be simply to list them and then introduce your activity. A balance has to be found between giving enough information to start people thinking, and giving too much information which then steers their thinking in a particular way. You may find it helpful to take Reflective Activity 1.1 above and adapt it as an introductory activity using your own words and style. Given the similarity of the ways in which spirituality and sexuality can be approached or avoided by healthcare professionals, it may add depth to your session if you include a brief comment or activity on sexuality.

At the end of each chapter you will find a section for the chaplain or spiritual care professional. These sections should enable you to develop and add depth to your personal understanding and self-awareness of spirituality.

FURTHER READING

Browse the shelves of the professional journals in your local healthcare library for articles on spirituality or spiritual care, or conduct a literature search using the term 'spiritual' to see how the authors' understanding of spirituality agrees or differs.

REFERENCES

1 UK Board of Healthcare Chaplaincy. *Spiritual and Religious Care Capabilities and Competences for Healthcare Chaplains.* Cambridge: UK Board of Healthcare Chaplaincy; 2009.
2 The Scottish Government. *Chief Executive Letter (2008) 49 – Spiritual Care.* Edinburgh: The Scottish Government Healthcare Policy and Strategy Directorate; 2008.

CHAPTER 2

Faith, belief and culture

INTRODUCTION

In healthcare, the quality strategy of advanced care planning encourages us to adopt a person-centred approach to care.[1] If healthcare is to focus on the individual, then by its very nature that should include our individual faith, beliefs and culture, whatever they might be – religious, secular or a blend of both. There is a small but vocal voice of opinion that states faith and belief should be separated from the institutions and services of state such as the National Health Service (NHS).[2] The authors believe that this view misunderstands the inherent influence of faith, belief and culture in all human beings.

In considering the value and influence of faith, belief and culture, the authors support the following inclusive definitions of the NHS and the UK Board of Healthcare Chaplaincy (UKBHC).[3–6]

➤ **Faith community:** *a recognisable group who share a belief system and usually undertake religious practices such as prayer, scripture reading, meditation and communal acts of worship.*

➤ **Belief group:** *any group which has a cohesive system of values or beliefs, but which does not classify itself as a faith community.*

These definitions acknowledge and distinguish the religious and humanist perspectives, yet enable them to stand alongside each other and work together. Indeed many of the national guidelines, standards and documents have been positively influenced by the inclusion of the Humanist Society as a recognised belief group.

It is also worth noting the definition of what is meant by an 'individual', as this demonstrates the inclusive nature of this topic and the focus of this book.

➤ **Individual:** *any person ... including: patients, service users, clients, relatives, carers, and NHS staff, or groups thereof.*

This chapter will enable the reader to explore the influence of faith, belief and culture in our personal and professional life. As in Chapter 1, self-awareness is the key, and reflecting on our own understanding and experiences will earth our understanding and the influence of faith, belief and culture in those we seek to care for. A person-centred approach to care rather than an in-depth study of the various world religions and belief systems is the way to best practice.

THE MEANING OF HEALTH

The German theologian, Paul Tillich, emphasises in the human condition the deep longing for being 'whole, not yet split, not disrupted, not disintegrated, and therefore healthy and sane'.[7]

Healthcare is thus fundamentally an activity that enables people to re-establish a whole that was broken. In many instances this means making new or broader connections to a reality that may have to include illness and suffering, the success or failure of treatment, and even dying, death and bereavement. To be healthy, therefore, is to be completely related or (inter)connected to the psyche, society, the cosmos, and the reality that we face.

Within this context of a return to wholeness, some will process their desire for healing through religious beliefs or practices. Religion, in its best sense, means 'to be connected', arising as it does from the Latin word *religare*, meaning 'to bind together into one bundle or sheaf'. Not surprisingly, therefore, the influence of faith, belief and culture remains important for many people as professional and personal frameworks seek to provide environments in which broken people find that they can be 'bound together' again, and reconnected to the things that matter to them.

PERSON-CENTRED APPROACH

A person-centred approach, while it is the ideal in healthcare, becomes essential when we seek to include faith, belief and culture in our assessment and care. The following section on faith, belief and culture will consider the complexity of caring for individuals who may self-identify and say that they adhere to a particular religion or belief group, yet in life and living show considerable variety in their beliefs and practices.

The only way to truly understand an individual's beliefs and practices, and what impact these may have on care for that patient and their carers, is to conduct an individual assessment. This is explored further in Chapter 6, on disentangling spiritual and religious care.

FAITH AND BELIEF

Each religion has its own clearly defined set of beliefs and practices that differ from each other and distinguish the different world religions. However, within each of these distinguishing religious labels, such as Buddhism, Christianity, Islam, Judaism and Sikhism, are a host of different denominations, schools or branches. Each of these branches will differ in their interpretation of the main principles, beliefs and practices of their religion. Furthermore, within each of these branches there are local faith communities and belief groups that may differ in yet other ways, and are influenced by local customs and cultures. Finally, within local faith communities and belief groups are the individuals who increasingly choose what elements of their faith community or belief group they will personally adhere to and practise. Members of faith communities and belief groups, like those with no formal religious association, can also adopt a 'pick and mix' approach to their understanding of faith and belief.

In addition to this variety of individual beliefs, many religions make exemptions from certain religious practices for the sick and those who are frail. However, each individual can choose whether to use the exemption or ignore it.

The following case scenario highlights the necessity for a person-centred approach to faith and belief, rather than relying on our assumed knowledge and experience of caring for individuals from recognised faith communities or belief groups.

Case Scenario 2.1

On entering the ward to visit his mother, Mr Mansur is approached by his mother's named nurse, John, who informs him that his mother is comfortable although not communicating. Having cared for an elderly Muslim patient before, John has arranged a Halal meal at lunchtime, has arranged for a female doctor, and is looking into the possibility of asking an interpreter to try to help with communication.

However, Mr Mansur is quiet but clearly distressed. His mother is in fact Hindu, a strict vegetarian, has no issues with gender, and uses English as her first language. She has been admitted with a urinary tract infection, which is why she appears confused and is having difficulty communicating.

Although in this case John was unable to 'ask the person' about their faith and beliefs, it is also clear that his assumptions based on his past experience caused distress to the patient's family. Although healthcare professionals who are seeking to assess the faith, belief and cultural elements of spiritual care can benefit from a general understanding of the main world faiths that are present in their local area, it is clear that an individual person-centred approach is essential.

To help to raise staff awareness of the likely faith and belief needs of patients, you may find that you have a local Multi-Faith Guide in your hospital or UK Department of Health. One comprehensive guide is *A Multi-Faith Resource for Healthcare Staff*.[8]

The resource book gives basic advice for the main faith communities and belief groups in the UK, and considers attitudes and practices in the following areas:

➤ birth customs
➤ death customs

➤ religious practices
➤ food and fasting
➤ washing and toilet
➤ modesty and dress
➤ family planning
➤ blood transfusions and organ donations.

The following activity will help you to consider your personal beliefs and practices and to explore to what degree you adhere to the beliefs and practices of the faith community or belief group with which you identify yourself. It will also enable you to reflect on how your personal beliefs might affect your professional practice.

Reflective Activity 2.1

Access a copy of your local Multi-Faith Guide or download a copy of *A Multi-Faith Resource for Healthcare Staff,*[8] and look up the section that relates to your personal faith community or belief group. If you do not identify yourself with a particular faith community or belief group, read the section on humanism.

Note down those elements that:
• reflect your personal beliefs and attitudes
• differ from your personal beliefs and attitudes.

What would this mean for you as a professional who is caring for people who say that they subscribe to the same faith community or belief group as you, yet on assessment differ in their beliefs and practices?

With this insight into and awareness of your own faith or beliefs, the following activity will enable you to explore faith and belief groups that differ from your own. In preparation for this activity you may find it helpful to think of the faith or belief groups that you regularly encounter in your workplace.

Reflective Activity 2.2

Return to your Multi-Faith Guide and choose a faith community or belief group that differs from your own, and note the beliefs and practices that differ from yours.

If you were caring for a patient or their family/carers from this particular faith community or belief group:
• What implications for practice would you identify for your work setting?
• What would be the difficulties and how might they be overcome?

You can repeat this activity for all faith communities and belief groups with which you regularly come into contact.

These activities and the multi-faith guidelines serve as a basic introduction to the topic of faith and belief. They are useful as a guide when we are faced with caring for a patient whom we know little about, as in Case Scenario 2.1 above, and can help us to avoid making mistaken basic assumptions that can cause offence or distress. The considerable individual variety in the way in which people practise their faith or beliefs means that the only effective assessment is a person-centred approach, so *ask the person*, or if they are unable to communicate, ask their family or carers.

CULTURE

The UK is described as a multicultural and multi-faith society. When considering faith and belief, the term 'multi-faith' can be used to describe the range of faith communities and belief groups that exist in society, as outlined above. However, it can also be interpreted as referring to a society where individuals do not adhere to one particular faith community or belief group, but rather feel able to 'pick and mix' from different faiths and beliefs. This means that rather than society simply becoming more atheist or secular in nature and rejecting long-held religious values, the variety of spiritual beliefs and cultural norms is increasing.

Different cultures are usually influenced by religious morality, beliefs and practices. For example, with regard to its laws, customs and holidays, the UK is influenced by Judaeo-Christian traditions. These often have their roots in attitudes, beliefs and practices that were prevalent so long ago that the people who belong to that culture today may fail to understand the religious and moral connection. As with faith and belief, culture will also be diverse and vary from one individual to another.

An individual's culture can be influenced by:
➤ his or her sense of nationality
➤ local customs and practices
➤ the family in which he or she grew up
➤ any faith community or belief group that is recognised as significant
➤ his or her peer group of friends.

Not surprisingly, the possible permutations within this list of influences lead to considerable diversity, even within normally clearly defined and understood cultural groups. As with spirituality, faith and belief, the only true understanding of a person's culture will come from a person-centred approach – *ask the person*.

WHAT DOES THIS MEAN FOR HEALTHCARE PRACTICE?

An understanding of the reality of a multicultural and multi-faith society has significant implications for health and social care professionals. As outlined above, society is becoming more diverse, as people 'pick and mix' what they believe and practise from the traditional faith communities, belief groups and cultural values. However, what people cannot turn away from are the attitudes, anxieties, aspirations, hopes and fears in the cultural and spiritual domain that are a natural part of health, well-being, illness, dying and death.

Although self-awareness of our own personal faith, beliefs and culture is helpful in providing a basis for our understanding of others, it also raises the possibility of caring for people who have values and practices that differ from and sometimes conflict with our own (*see* Chapter 9). However, it is also true that many patients and their family/carers ask questions of healthcare professionals that call on us to integrate our personal and professional lives.

Should you share what you believe?

While a personal understanding of our own faith, belief and culture gives us a context from which to assess and explore the needs of patients and their carers, there is a balance to be found between our personal and professional roles. 'Should you share what you believe?' is a particularly pertinent question when our personal faith, beliefs and values are strong and deeply held.

There are two basic guidelines to follow when considering whether to share what we believe with patients and their family/carers:

➤ Has the patient asked you what you believe?
➤ Will your words be supportive to the patient?

The following case scenario gives an example.

CASE SCENARIO 2.2

Janice is a 50-year-old primary school headteacher. She is in the end stages of acute myeloid leukaemia, and for the past two weeks has been a patient in the hospital. She is a deeply religious woman whose Christian faith is an important sustaining feature for her in her end-of-life journey. She has a supportive pastor from her church, and many friends who come to visit, some of whom pray with her and read the Bible to her. She has several religious artefacts around her bed-space. In the early hours one morning, when Janice is unable to sleep, she confides to one of the night staff that she is frightened that she's 'not been good enough', and that God might be angry with her. The nurse asks her if she has been 'baptised in the spirit'. Janice says she doesn't understand what this means, and is told that it's a 'second baptism', and that people who have not experienced it won't get to heaven. Janice affirms that she was baptised as a baby, and asks 'Isn't that enough?' The response is that it is not, and that heaven only welcomes those who have had a 'spirit-baptism' in their adult life.

Taking this scenario at face value we could debate whether or not the patient was indirectly asking what the nurse believed, or whether the nurse's words were supportive. That discussion in itself would miss the point of what the patient is saying. The key sentence is in the patient's statement that '… *she is frightened that she's "not been good enough", and that God might be angry with her.*'

The following activity will help you to think through what response you might give to a similar patient.

Reflective Activity 2.3

From Case Scenario 2.2, a patient who presents as a deeply religious person appears to be experiencing fear, is questioning her faith and beliefs and is worried about the anger of God.

What would be your response to the patient statement: '*I'm frightened that I've not been good enough, and that God might be angry with me*'?

There is no one correct response, and each of the following would be appropriate:
➤ Reflect the statement back to the patient and seek to explore their feelings.
➤ Acknowledge to the patient that you don't feel you have the experience and/ or knowledge to think through these issues and with the patient's permission:
  – refer them on to another member of the team with more skill in this area
  – refer them on to a chaplain.

This case scenario and activity is another example where the answer to the question that is being asked will be less important than finding out why the question is being asked in the first place. In Chapter 12 we shall look at ways in which chaplaincy services can be used to help us to build our experience in this area of care.

This chapter has sought to guide us through the complexities of faith, belief and culture in the world in which we live. From a position of self-awareness of our attitudes and beliefs with regard to life, living, health, dying and death, we can then journey with others. In seeking to assess and address spiritual needs that are influenced by an individual's faith belief and culture, we enter into an area of increasing diversity. Yet complex as this whole area is, there is a very simple solution – focus on the individual, apply the principles of person-centred care and remember to *ask the person*.

CHAPLAIN OR SPIRITUAL CARE PROFESSIONAL

Religion, faith and belief are the area of expertise of the chaplain or spiritual care professional. However, the same criteria of self-awareness apply. It is for this reason that all chaplains who are registered with the UK Board of Healthcare Chaplaincy must maintain a recognised status in a mainstream faith community or belief group.[9] It is the in-depth personal experience of faith and belief that enables the chaplain to journey with others into the variety of individual beliefs and experiences.

Although it is helpful for all healthcare professionals to have a measure of insight into the different faith communities and belief groups, for the chaplain it is essential. Chaplaincy services should have established relationships with the faith communities in their local area and have a readily available list of contacts for healthcare staff to consult and use.[10]

The chaplain's role in responding to the more complex issues of faith, belief and culture will vary. It may entail offering advice to support the other healthcare professionals who are involved with service users, or it may be that their direct involvement by referral is most appropriate, as in Reflective Activity 2.3 above.

The following activity will encourage you to reflect on a complex case scenario and to consider what issues you foresee arising and how you might resolve them.

CASE SCENARIO 2.3

A patient on the ward has just died, and nursing staff have made an urgent referral to which you respond. The referral included the following information. The patient is Muslim and Egyptian. His wife and son are with him, and the patient's brother is due to arrive to make arrangements to have the patient's body repatriated to Egypt for burial.

On speaking with his wife you discover that she and her 17-year-old stepson are Christian, white and UK nationals. She wants to have her husband buried in his home country, as he requested. However, her son does not have a passport and she is worried that there will not be enough time to obtain one.

While you are with the family the nurse asks to speak with you. When speaking to the contracted funeral director she was informed that the body will need to be embalmed before air travel. It is recorded in the patient notes that the patient had hepatitis C, and the funeral director says that this is a problem, as their health and safety guidelines do not permit their staff to embalm bodies that have hepatitis C.

Reflective Activity 2.4

Reflecting on the above case scenario, what are the main concerns you would have about the situation and the different members of the family? How would you seek to resolve those concerns?

You may find the following list a helpful starting point.
- Can a passport/visa for a 17-year-old be arranged at short notice?
- What is the law on repatriation of remains by air?
- Does the patient's wife know that the patient had hepatitis C?
- Will there be specific religious or cultural needs at this time and, if so, who would be best placed to meet them?

A chaplain who works in an area of care where the repatriation of remains abroad is a regular occurrence will build up a wealth of experience. That experience can be a valuable resource for others for whom this will be a rare yet (when it happens) pressing problem.

This chapter has sought to outline the complexities of faith, belief and culture as they arise in what is termed our multi-faith, multicultural society. This area of care is one that forms part of the expertise and specialism that is healthcare chaplaincy. We need to know where we are rooted if we are to be able to journey with others through the complexities and individual variety of faith, belief and culture, yet the same simple person-centred approach still applies – *ask the person.*

FURTHER READING

➤ Consult your local multi-faith or multicultural guide.
➤ Consult your list of local and national contacts for faith community and belief group leaders.
➤ NHS Education for Scotland. *A Multi-Faith Resource for Healthcare Staff.* Glasgow: NHS Education for Scotland Healthcare Chaplaincy Training and Development Unit; 2006.

REFERENCES

1   e-Learning for Healthcare (e-LfH). *Individual, Cultural and Spiritual Influences Within the Context of Advanced Care Planning.* London: Department of Health. www.e-lfh.org.uk (accessed February 2010).
2   National Secular Society. *An Investigation into the Cost of the National Health Service's Chaplaincy Provision.* London: National Secular Society. www.secularism.org.uk (accessed December 2010).
3   UK Board of Healthcare Chaplaincy. *Standards for NHS Chaplaincy Services.* Cambridge: UK Board of Healthcare Chaplaincy; 2009.
4   UK Board of Healthcare Chaplaincy. *Spiritual and Religious Care Capabilities and Competences for Healthcare Chaplains.* Cambridge: UK Board of Healthcare Chaplaincy; 2009.
5   NHS Education for Scotland. *Spiritual and Religious Care Capabilities and Competences for Healthcare Chaplains.* Edinburgh: NHS Education for Scotland; 2008.
6   Association of Hospice and Palliative Care Chaplains (AHPCC), College of Health Care Chaplains (CHCC) and Scottish Association of Chaplains in Healthcare (SACH). *Standards for NHS Scotland Chaplaincy Services.* Glasgow: AHPCC, CHCC, SACH, and NHS Education for Scotland Healthcare Chaplaincy Training and Development Unit; 2007.
7   Tillich P. *The Relation of Religion and Health: historical considerations and theological questions.* Cited by Grau K. Salvation as cosmic healer in Tillich. *North American Paul Tillich Society Newsletter* 2002; **28**: 24.

8 NHS Education for Scotland. *A Multi-Faith Resource for Healthcare Staff*. Glasgow: NHS Education for Scotland Healthcare Chaplaincy Training and Development Unit; 2006.

9 UK Board of Healthcare Chaplaincy. *Spiritual and Religious Care Capabilities and Competences for Healthcare Chaplains*, op. cit.

10 UK Board of Healthcare Chaplaincy. *Standards for NHS Chaplaincy Services*, op. cit.

CHAPTER 3

Communication issues and skills

INTRODUCTION

Having already considered our self-awareness of spirituality and the ways in which it can be provided and by whom, we now turn to another core element of spiritual care, namely communication. For good spiritual care to take place, healthcare professionals need to develop good interpersonal skills. Core to this skill-set are communication skills.

Good interpersonal communication has long been seen as a core skill for healthcare professionals. The National Institute for Clinical Excellence notes that:

> Interpersonal communication is the process of information exchange among patients, carers and health and social care professionals. It is underpinned and enhanced by mutual understanding, respect and awareness of individuals' roles and functions, and is the process through which patients and carers are helped to explore issues and arrive at decisions.[1]

However, when we consider communication alongside spiritual care, we go beyond information giving and are firmly rooted in the 'personal' part of 'interpersonal.' Here the quality of the therapeutic relationship matters, as does the healthcare professional's ability to relate at a personal as well as a professional level. Again this is not new, and the Department of Health notes that the humanity and personal facets of healthcare professionals make a difference:

> Research evidence indicates that a 'willingness to listen and explain' is considered by patients to be one of the essential attributes of a health professional (along with sensitivity, approachability, respect and honesty).[2]

This chapter will consider the context of communication in spiritual care and then encourage the reader to reflect on the communication skills that can be developed and enhanced to enable the delivery of competent and good spiritual care.

COMMUNICATION IN THE CONTEXT OF SPIRITUAL CARE

Communication in the context of spiritual care has two significant elements. The first element consists of the interpersonal skills, and ways of using these skills to facilitate good spiritual care. However, the second element is the uncomfortable one, where we realise that the context for using our communication skills is bound up with what we would normally term the patient's private life.

As noted in Chapter 5, when our competency in spiritual care increases, so does the depth of spiritual care that we find ourselves dealing with. This depth or complexity usually arises from the fact that spiritual care (or, more importantly, spiritual need or spiritual distress) often has its roots in ethical, moral, spiritual, religious or existential issues rather than our area of clinical expertise. The terrifying 'Why?' questions to which there are no hard-and-fast answers are one example of the depth of spiritual care.

The principle of self-awareness outlined in Chapter 1 also applies here. If we are to enter into the spiritual domain of people's lives, we need to have insight into, and an understanding of, what we believe about these same issues to enable us to safely journey with others and explore their spiritual needs and distress.

The following activities will help you to begin that journey by exploring the impact of ethical, moral, spiritual, religious and existential issues in your workplace setting.

Reflective Activity 3.1

> Reflect on your own workplace setting and the patients and their family/carers who are under your care. Make a note of what draws you to that area of care. What are the elements of the work that make it worthwhile for you?
>
> Make a second list of the moral, ethical, spiritual or existential questions or issues that you come to experience and have to deal with.

Most healthcare professionals when reflecting in this way find that their own personal beliefs are naturally aligned with the care setting in which they work. This is not surprising, since for many healthcare professionals a strong element of their personal spirituality comes from their work and the satisfaction and meaning that they draw from it. However, these same positive understandings, beliefs and experiences can often help us to understand why there are other areas of care with which we are not so comfortable.

The following activity will help you to explore what areas of care you might find difficult to work in, and why.

Reflective Activity 3.2

From your experience, reflect on an area of care in which you know from experience or feel from instinct that you would not choose to work.

Make a note of what it is that would make it difficult for you, or what you would dislike or feel uncomfortable with.

Now reflect on the moral, ethical, spiritual or existential questions or issues that you feel you might find difficult or uncomfortable.

In completing these activities you will probably find that there is good reason why you find yourself working where you do with the patient group for whom you provide care. We naturally self-select a care setting in which we will feel comfortable, and although there will always be challenges, we start from a base where we have an understanding of the main issues and dilemmas. This is a strength, and it gives us a head start in dealing with the spiritual issues and difficult questions that we might find ourselves confronted with.

SKILLS IN COMMUNICATION

The core skills for communication in spiritual care are no different from those in other areas of healthcare. Listening would come top of a long list that includes acknowledgement, encouragement, using open questions, picking up cues, reflection and clarification.

Reflective Activity 3.3

Reflect on a typical scenario from your own clinical experience which you find challenging or uncomfortable, and where you had to have an in-depth conversation with a patient or their family/carers.

Complete the following self-assessment table by considering whether or not in your regular communication you use these skills, and for those skills that you do use, grade yourself on your ability.

Communication skill	Is this a skill that you use?	Self-assessment (on a scale of 1–5)
Ask one question at a time		
Use open questions		
Use clarification to check your own understanding		
Use reflection		

(continued)

Communication skill	Is this a skill that you use?	Self-assessment (on a scale of 1–5)
Control the pace and direction of the interview sensitively		
Follow relevant cues		
Use silence appropriately		

The use of open questions, the following of relevant cues and the appropriate use of silence are the most useful skills when starting a spiritual conversation/assessment. The other skills are used to add depth and gain understanding. The depth of spiritual care that we are able to offer will also depend on the relationship that we have with the individual and their perception of the human qualities we embody, such as respect, honesty and listening.

The following section of this chapter will consider the use and development of these skills in providing spiritual care.

CHALLENGES IN COMMUNICATION

The most significant challenge to communication in spiritual care is ourselves. As human beings and healthcare professionals we are wary of causing offence, hurt or embarrassment, and since by its very nature spiritual care can involve exploring what we consider to be an individual's personal or private life, we are naturally wary and on guard.

The way in which spiritual issues are raised can also be a challenge. Patients will often choose carefully who they will raise significant issues with. It may be a nurse whom they see regularly and with whom they have developed a good relationship. However, it is just as likely to be the healthcare assistant during the intimacy of a bath, or a physiotherapist or occupational therapist whom they will only see occasionally. They might also sound out different people to see if they get the same response.

The ways in which spiritual issues surface are commonly indirect, and we need good communication skills to get beneath the surface. The challenges can arise through difficult questions, strong emotions and collusion.

The following sections will consider each of these areas and how we might use communication skills to work through them.

Responding to difficult questions

What constitutes a difficult question will depend on our individual experience. What makes it difficult is whether or not we have an answer to the question.

Often in the case of the difficult spiritual questions there is no answer to the question.

Read the following case scenarios and decide which would be a 'difficult question' for you.

CASE SCENARIO 3.1

John is being accompanied on a home assessment visit by an occupational therapist and a nurse. It is three months since he was last home, and his mobility, although recently improved, is not as good as it was before. He is unable to manage the stairs to his bedroom, but the bathroom is downstairs, and the family have converted the lounge into a bedroom/ sitting room. John is asked what he thinks of the changes and in reply asks you: 'Am I dying?'

CASE SCENARIO 3.2

Two weeks ago Roberta was on the golf course with her friends playing her regular daily round. She went to the doctor with an intermittent pain in her back and is now bedbound and cannot walk. You are hoisting Roberta into the bath and she exclaims: 'This is so unfair, why has this happened to me? Tell me what have I done to deserve this.'

CASE SCENARIO 3.3

Danny is 14 years old and has been re-admitted to the ward after a second suicide attempt. His dad, George, found him at home and was able to get the paramedics in time. Danny has been sedated and George is sitting by his bedside and begins to tell you the story of the family. He says Danny took it hard when his big brother was murdered and it was Danny who found him. Danny's mum never got over it either and died just a few months ago. George stops talking for a few minutes, then turns and looks you in the eye and asks: 'Why is it that some people get so much to bear? What kind of God is it that would allow these things to happen?'

Regardless of whether you find that one or all of these scenarios present difficult questions, the key to responding to them is the same. When we are dealing with these big *'Why?'* questions, we need to begin by understanding that the question itself is rarely important. Instead it is the cue to something else. We are not expected to try and answer the *'Why?'* questions. Instead we need to find out why the question is being asked.

It is here that the core communication skills are useful, namely the use of open questions, the following of cues and the appropriate use of silence. Open questions (i.e. questions to which there is no 'yes' or 'no' answer) are particularly useful for engaging in deep conversations. They encourage the individual to talk, and will elicit the cues we are looking for to get behind the initial question. As these are often weighty answers, people sometimes need some time to think. Here silence is a good tool for giving the person time to think and respond.

In practice we can often use an open question as a stock answer that can turn the conversation around, and seek to follow the cue and find out what is behind the question. For example, in Case Scenarios 3.1, 3.2 and 3.3 above, an appropriate response might be: 'These are very deep questions. What's put them in your mind?' or 'That's one of those questions to which there is no easy answer. What's put that in your mind?'

Reflective Activity 3.4

> Re-read the three case scenarios above and think about how you would respond in each case. You might find it helpful to write down the actual words that you would use.

Responding to strong emotions

A common sign of spiritual distress is anger. Anger is a strong emotion, and it can be frightening and threatening to be confronted with it. Communication skills theory offers a framework for dealing with anger which includes the following:

➤ recognition (acknowledging that you realise the person is angry)
➤ permission (letting the person know that it is OK to be angry)
➤ listening to the story in order to obtain as much information as possible
➤ focusing on the individual's stress and/or other feelings.[3]

When responding to an angry person we need to see beyond the emotion and find its cause. Talking less and listening more is the best strategy. Again, the use of open questions and silence to allow the person to speak are often the most helpful skills.

The following case scenarios and activities will help you to reflect on your practice and identify a strategy for responding to anger.

CASE SCENARIO 3.4

Doreen has been admitted for end-of-life care and has stopped eating and drinking. Her daughter, Isobel, has just arrived from her home in Canada and is surprised at the deterioration in her mother since the last time she visited, which was 9 months ago. Isobel is standing at the foot of her mother's bed and in a very loud, forceful voice is addressing you: 'What kind of care are you offering here? Look at the state my mother is in. Where is the care? She's clearly dehydrated. Why is she not on a drip? Why is she not in a side room? This is appalling care. Who is in charge here? Who are you and what are you going to do about this?'

Isobel is clearly angry, and her anger appears to be focused on a number of practical issues. However, there could also be other underlying spiritual issues of which the anger is a symptom. The following activity will help you to think about how you might respond to Isobel and identify any underlying spiritual issues.

Reflective Activity 3.5

Reflecting on the anger that is being directed to you from Isobel in Case Scenario 3.4, how would you respond to her questions: *'What kind of care are you offering here? Look at the state my mother is in. Where is the care? She's clearly dehydrated. Why is she not on a drip? Why is she not in a side room? This is appalling care. Who is in charge here? Who are you and what are you going to do about this?'*
- Write down the first thing you would say to Isobel.
- Make a list of some open questions you might use to find out Isobel's story and assess any spiritual issues or distress.

There are no set answers for these situations. However, acknowledging the anger and combining this acknowledgement with open questions to show that you hear what the person is saying and are taking the situation seriously can help. For example, *'My name is Jan and I work on the ward. I can see that you are quite angry and I would like to help. What would you say is the most pressing thing you are angry about?'*

As with all communication issues, when anger is combined with the presence of other family or carers, the level of complexity increases significantly, as the continuing case scenario demonstrates.

CASE SCENARIO 3.4 CONTINUED

Having spent time with Isobel, you discover that she was taken completely by surprise at the change in her mother's appearance compared with the last time she had seen her. Isobel's brother, Brian, who looked after their mum, had been keeping things from Isobel to protect her.

Later that day you hear a loud commotion and you find Isobel and Brian standing on either side of their mother's bed having a loud argument about what should happen when their mother dies. Isobel is shouting: 'Mother made me promise that she would be cremated and not buried. She hated the thought of burial.' Brian is equally loud and adamant: 'Mum wanted to be buried with Dad. That was her wish and that's what's in her will.'

You are concerned for the other patients in the bay who are visibly distressed by the argument.

Reflective Activity 3.6

Reflecting on the continuing case scenario, which of the following would you do next?
- Ask the relatives to lower their voices?
- Take the relatives to a different room?
- Take the relatives to separate rooms?
- Call for help?
- Something else?

What would you say to try to bring about your choice of response? Write down the actual words you would use.

Families add a different dynamic to strong emotions such as anger. Often there will be deep-rooted issues underlying the argument. It is worth remembering that healthcare chaplains and social workers often have considerable skills and experience in dealing with complex family dynamics and disagreements. Although you will need a strategy to deal with the initial situation, it may be most appropriate for you to refer the family on, especially if you need to spend time with the patient.

Working through collusion

'Please don't tell my dad how bad it is or that it's cancer.'

Such a request is often the starting point on the road to collusion. Although there is no doubt that sometimes family or carers do know best, collusion is very difficult to maintain and uphold on the rare occasions when it is justified. These pleas are somewhat similar to the *'Why?'* questions that we explored above. They are a way of articulating some deep and often heartfelt anxiety, fear or spiritual distress.

Communication skills training can offer a structure for dealing with collusion that includes taking the request seriously, finding out the relative's reasons for asking, seeking permission to find out what the patient already knows, and giving reassurance that you will not provide information if you are not asked. However, as with the other challenges to communication that have already been explored, the underlying issues in collusion should be identified. This can be achieved by using open questions, picking up cues and listening. For example, a series of open questions in response to the plea *'Please don't tell my dad how bad it is or that it's cancer'* might include the following:

➤ What worries you most about your dad finding out?
➤ What kind of questions has your dad been asking recently?
➤ How does your dad usually deal with difficult news?

The following activity will help you to consider what you might say to get beyond the initial plea and open up the conversation.

Reflective Activity 3.7

> A patient accompanied by his daughter is being brought into your clinical area. Before the patient is brought in, his daughter makes a point of getting you on your own and then says: 'I need you to promise me that you won't tell my dad what he's got or how serious it is. It would destroy him.'
> - How would you respond?

As stated in the introduction to this chapter, the communication skills that are used in spiritual care are no different from those in which we are experienced in other areas of care. Core skills such as listening, acknowledgement, encouragement, using open questions, picking up cues, reflection and clarification are all useful. The complexity of communication in spiritual care arises from the complexity of our own anxiety and fears, and from the personal or private nature of the spiritual need or distress.

Rarely is the difficult question, the strong emotion or the request for collusion the main issue. Rather, these are often a means whereby the patient or carer is indicating that there is something significant underneath which they are finding difficult to get out or articulate. We each need a strategy to help us to cope. Sometimes the strategy will be to get beyond the surface and into the depth of why the question has been asked or why the person is so angry. However, sometimes we might need to recognise that we don't have time for this conversation or to separate the patient and their family. In this case, we need a strategy for referral and help. Good communication skills can enable us to find both and use them accordingly.

CHAPLAIN OR SPIRITUAL CARE PROFESSIONAL

Advanced communication skills are a core skill for healthcare chaplains. The case scenarios that have already been outlined in this chapter will often be referred to chaplaincy services because of their complexity and the nature of the questions that are being asked. Not surprisingly, the UK Board of Healthcare Chaplaincy has a specific capability and a number of competences in this area for chaplains:[4]

> 1.3. Communication skills: The chaplain maintains and develops the communication skills necessary for the spiritual and religious care of individuals and groups.

> Chaplains should demonstrate an ability to:
> > 1.3.1. use communication skills to provide pastoral care
> > 1.3.2. identify language needs and interpreting services
> > 1.3.3. communicate with individuals in a variety of complex encounters

1.3.4. contribute to interprofessional communication

1.3.5. maintain confidentiality and informed consent.

The most challenging competence in this list is communicating in complex pastoral encounters. It is here that the chaplain's communication skills need to be honed and used thoughtfully and creatively. The following case scenario highlights the complexity and often urgency of complex pastoral encounters, and the reflective activity that follows it will help you to consider the communication skills you could employ.

CASE SCENARIO 3.4 CONTINUED

As chaplain you receive an urgent call to the ward to deal with two angry relatives. You arrive and are told that the relatives were fighting over the patient and causing a commotion. There was only one relatives' room available and they have both been 'put' in there and the nurses are working with the other patients who were distressed by the commotion.

When you enter the room, Brian, the patient's son, stands up, turns to you and says: 'Thank God! Can you please help us sort this out? Mum told 'her' she wants to be cremated but she told me that she wants to be buried and that's what's in her will, so we have to do that, don't we?'

Before you can answer, Isobel, the patient's daughter, also stands up and turns to you and says: 'I can't take any more of this. This is a nightmare!'

Often in urgent and complex pastoral encounters such as this the chaplain can find him- or herself knowing very little of the situation before being confronted with the people involved and the raw emotions and heated questions. Although this is unnerving, it can also be a strength rather than a weakness, as it enables us to come afresh to the situation and to use the same communication skills as those outlined above – open questions, silence and following cues – to open a dialogue and get behind the emotions and distress.

The following reflective activity will help you to reflect on and develop your strategy for dealing with complex pastoral encounters.

Reflective Activity 3.8

Having read the continuation of Case Scenario 3.4 above, what would be your first response to the brother and sister who are standing before you?
• Write down the words you would say.

There may be a number of issues running through your head at this time – practical issues relating to cremation, burial, interment of ashes, whether or not you have to adhere to the wishes made in a will, who is next of kin, and who will have the death certificate and therefore have responsibility for the funeral. Although it may be tempting to unpick this jumble, is that really what this case scenario is about? In short, we don't know and we need to shelve these practical questions for now until we can get the whole story, and we need to bear in mind that the story may differ depending on whom we are talking to.

Reflective Activity 3.9

Assuming that you are going to shelve the practical questions until later, prepare a number of open questions that you might use to get behind the questions and emotions.

Depending on the responses to these questions, you might choose to work with the situation as it is with the brother and sister together, or you might choose to include a colleague and work with the siblings separately. Reflecting on your workplace setting, who would you refer them to who would have similar skills for dealing with complex communication issues?

Although all healthcare professionals can benefit from enhanced communication skills, these are a core skill for healthcare chaplains. The context of pastoral encounters, the difficult questions, the strong emotions and the differing views of family members and/or carers all contribute to the complexity of pastoral care. Developing enhanced communication skills is essential to enable us to respond to referrals, support patients and their family carers, and support our colleagues in the healthcare team.

FURTHER READING

Although a number of books are available to help individuals to reflect on their communication skills, the authors would encourage the reader to undertake an advanced communication skills course such as the Wilkinson and Roberts model.[5] Such courses allow us to practise and develop our skills in a real and safe way.

REFERENCES

1 National Institute for Clinical Excellence. *Improving Supportive and Palliative Care for Adults with Cancer. Manual.* London: National Institute for Clinical Excellence; 2004.
2 Department of Health. *The NHS Cancer Plan: a plan for investment, a plan for reform.* London: Department of Health; 2000.
3 UK Board of Healthcare Chaplaincy. *Spiritual and Religious Care Capabilities and Competences for Healthcare Chaplains.* Cambridge: UK Board of Healthcare Chaplaincy; 2009.
4 Wilkinson S, Roberts A. *Communication Skills Course.* London: Marie Curie Cancer Care; 2004.
5 Wilkinson S, Roberts A. *Communication Skills Course,* op. cit.

CHAPTER 4

The healthcare team

INTRODUCTION

If spiritual care is to be assessed and responded to appropriately at all levels of competency in a holistic healthcare context, the role, purpose and cohesion of the healthcare team are crucial. There is evidence that multi-disciplinary teams, particularly in specialist settings, improve patient satisfaction and deal more effectively with patient and family needs.[1] In addition, where care planning is facilitated in a team context not only is this more beneficial to the patient, but also it provides a clearer context in which journeys of care can be identified and examined from the perspective of the team, the patient and their carers.[2] In the field of mental health, for example, the process standards indicate that, in the team context, staff can begin to see where changes or improvements could be made by identifying gaps, overlaps, strengths and weaknesses in the delivery of care. This leads to good teamworking, the development of shared goals and responsibilities, and an improvement in the care that is being offered.

As was pointed out in the previous chapter, not every healthcare setting will have a clear understanding of a team approach to healthcare, or access to a variety of professional roles, far less individuals who might operate at different levels of competency. Some healthcare professionals work either exclusively or for long periods as lone practitioners (e.g. a district nurse in a remote rural setting, or a community palliative care nurse on night shift). For such lone practitioners, access to teamworking with opportunities to meet with and take advice from colleagues can be very limited.

The following definition of a multi-disciplinary healthcare team and Reflective Activity 4.1 will encourage the reader to reflect on the size and composition of the healthcare team(s) of which they are a part.

The Clinical Standards Board for Scotland and the Scottish Partnership for Palliative Care in their *Clinical Standards for Specialist Palliative Care* make a distinction between the 'core team' in a specialist setting and 'access to' a wider team of healthcare professionals.[3]

The core team comprises dedicated sessional input from:

➤ chaplain
➤ doctors
➤ nurses
➤ occupational therapist
➤ pharmacist
➤ physiotherapist
➤ social worker.

There is ready access to other professionals including: anaesthetist (who is a specialist in pain management), bereavement specialists, complementary therapists, dentist, dietitian, lymphoedema specialists, oncologists, psychiatrists, psychologist and/or counsellor, speech and language therapist.

These additional professions can be termed the wider healthcare team.

Reflective Activity 4.1

Reflecting on the Clinical Standards Board definition of the core team above, and from your own experience:
• What professionals make up the core team in your care setting?
• What other professions would you have ready access to as the wider healthcare team?
• If you are a member of a number of healthcare teams, in which of these are you a core member of the team?

The composition of the team we have identified will depend on our profession and clinical setting. It might be a core team of doctors and nurses with others as the wider healthcare team, or it may be more multi-professional. As an allied health professional working across a number of teams you might consider yourself to be a core member of some teams but not others.

This chapter will take a team-based setting as the norm. In so doing, it will make no distinction between primary and secondary care, or distinguish between different healthcare settings (e.g. acute, mental health, paediatrics, palliative care, etc.). It will be for the reader to apply the information in this chapter to the healthcare setting in which they are particularly engaged, or of which they have detailed knowledge, and extrapolate to other settings which are not specifically touched upon.

TEAMWORKING

In exploring the palliative care context, Tebbit contends that a multi-professional team provides physical, psychological, social and spiritual support, and will provide practitioners with a broad mix of skills.[4] If spiritual care matters in all healthcare contexts and not just the specialist environments, a multi-professional context for the assessment and delivery of appropriate spiritual care is crucial. Such a multi-professional context assumes that:

➤ there are a variety of people engaged with patients and their carers at different levels of service delivery
➤ there are levels of competency which can be understood and developed
➤ there are referral criteria which offer guidance when issues are identified that challenge the boundaries of professional competence.

However, this will only work adequately if a team is in place and it functions well. Four things matter in this context:

1. Professional roles and responsibilities within the team should be clearly defined and understood by other team members.
2. In this regard, boundaries to levels of competency in the delivery of spiritual and religious care should be explored, agreed and understood by all members of the team. This should include clear guidance on the issue of confidentiality.
3. Referral criteria and methodologies for referrals also have to be worked through. They must be clearly understood and appropriately utilised by all members of the team. This should include standards and practices for appropriate recording.
4. The team should have regular opportunities for meeting together to explore the above, to further develop good working practices and to examine ways in which relationships within the team can be enhanced.

PROFESSIONAL ROLES AND RESPONSIBILITIES

It is easy – and dangerous – to assume that professional roles are always clearly understood by other healthcare professionals. It is important, therefore, that professional roles and responsibilities within a multi-professional team are clearly defined and understood by other team members.

For example, a physiotherapist 'does' physiotherapy. But what is that? What does it entail? We may assume that its purpose is to rehabilitate a patient, to help with mobility. But what actually happens? What techniques are utilised, and why? What training underpins professional practice? What are a physiotherapist's professional standards? What does it mean to be 'registered'? When is it appropriate to refer someone for physiotherapy? And if a patient confides in us that they are apprehensive of the 'physio-terrorist', does our ignorance of the *actual* role and expected outcomes further reinforce our own stereotypes and, unwittingly or not, support the patient in theirs? Similar questions arise when we make assumptions about or remain ignorant of the roles and responsibilities of an occupational therapist, a pharmacist, a dietitian, a chaplain, or any healthcare professional.

Such assumptions, ignorance, and resorting to or reinforcing stereotypes are dangerous in practice, both for the working of the team, and ultimately for the well-being of the patient.

The following Case Scenario and Reflective Activity will encourage you to consider the boundaries of your professional role and spiritual care.

CASE SCENARIO 4.1

Brenda is the physiotherapist on a stroke rehabilitation ward. She is working closely with Alex, aged 81 years, who has a right-sided weakness and slight dysphasia after a recent stroke. This is his third stroke in the past year, and he is struggling with his impaired mobility and inability to speak clearly. He is overwhelmed with a severe loss of confidence. After some exercises, Brenda is settling Alex back into his chair when he starts to cry. Brenda kneels down beside him and asks him what's wrong. It takes Alex a while to compose himself and communicate clearly. Eventually Brenda can make out the following words: 'It's the wife ...'

Reflective Activity 4.2

From your own professional experience, answer the following questions in relation to Case Scenario 4.1:
- Should Brenda have been concerned about Alex's emotions if her professional role was to attend to his physical needs?
- Why might Alex have chosen to confide in Brenda?
- What might Brenda do with what the information that emerges in Alex's story?
- How long should Brenda spend with Alex when there are many other patients to see to and further professional responsibilities to fulfil?

Any of the following assumptions (and many more besides) could be made by a passing chaplain, or any other healthcare professional, on seeing Brenda kneeling before a weeping patient:
➤ this is not her role
➤ she has made Alex cry, and therefore has done something inappropriate
➤ she is entering territory that rightly belongs to someone else – perhaps even you
➤ she is good at what she is doing
➤ Alex is confiding in her to slight you ...

Such might be the tensions that are experienced by you as a member of the team. If they are not dealt with and 'sorted' in an appropriate way, this can ultimately be detrimental to your own relationship with Brenda as a professional colleague, and consequently to the well-being of the whole team.

These tensions, and the suspicions, professional jealousies and reinforced stereotypes that may accompany them, can be more than adequately dissipated by a clearer understanding of each professional's roles and responsibilities. Would it not be useful for Brenda to explain to those who are not aware of this what rehabilitation after a stroke is seeking to achieve, what emotions are likely to be stirred up after a stroke, and how she handles these emotions when they arise? Might that not make for both a better understanding of her role, and a better working relationship with her?

Reflective Activity 4.3 will help you to explore the stereotypes related to the provision of spiritual care in particular.

Reflective Activity 4.3

From your own experience in the healthcare setting in which you have worked:
- What are the stereotypes that exist relating to chaplains and the delivery of spiritual care?
- To overcome these stereotypes, what questions would you ask a chaplain?
- If you are a chaplain, what might you usefully share with the rest of the team about your role and responsibilities?

PROFESSIONAL BOUNDARIES

It is, of course, clear enough that a patient will choose to confide in anyone whom they select. That is their right. This is the nature of good relationships built up between the patient and the healthcare professional. Often it will not be for the team member to choose whether a patient raises an issue. Brenda in Case Scenario 4.1 may have preferred Alex *not* to go into areas that were beyond the physical, or if he made comments or answered questions, she might have preferred that they should only be related to the physiotherapy input and what might be assumed to be solely her area of professional competence. However, for a tearful stroke patient, or a distressed patient at two o'clock in the morning, or someone being bathed or having a dressing changed, things will come up – whether the healthcare professional likes it or not. It is how that issue is responded to, and how subsequent issues are dealt with, that will define the efficacy of the encounter on behalf of the whole team, and ultimately whether the outcome is to the benefit of the patient's overall well-being and holistic care. This is all the more reason why, in this regard, boundaries to levels of competency in the delivery of spiritual and religious care have to be explored and understood by all members of the team, and this should include clear guidance on the issue of confidentiality.

Case Scenario 4.1 continues below, and is followed by Reflective Activity 4.4. This encourages you to move towards a deeper consideration of Alex's spiritual needs.

CASE SCENARIO 4.1 CONTINUED

Brenda encourages Alex to continue with his story and express his concerns. This process is slow and difficult. It would be too disruptive to take Alex to a private room so the conversation has to continue while lunch trolleys are moved around. In addition, a patient is in distress on the other side of the ward, a porter arrives with a wheelchair to take the patient in the next bed to X-ray and a nurse asks several times 'Are you done yet?', as it's time to help Alex with his lunch. And Brenda is more than aware that she had promised to meet someone 20 minutes ago. Alex tells her that he's frightened he might die. He has been his wife's main carer, and since his stroke she has had to stay in a care facility. They have no family, and there is no one 'to look after things'. Alex hasn't been able to visit his wife. He has no idea what is happening to her. He is worried about what the future will be for her after he's gone. He has not made plans for his funeral, and is not sure who will pay for it. He feels that he has let his wife down.

Reflective Activity 4.4

Reflecting on the development in the continuation of Case Scenario 4.1 above, consider the following questions:
* Would you consider Alex to be in spiritual distress? If so, what is the nature of that distress?
* How might Brenda respond to the issues that Alex has raised?
* What might be the actions that would follow this conversation?
* What outcomes might Brenda expect from this encounter which could be seen as being beneficial to Alex's well-being and helping to alleviate his spiritual distress?

Clearly, Alex has chosen this moment to flag up his emotional and spiritual concerns. And he has chosen this person with whom to share his deeper feelings and fears. Brenda could, of course, have given a clear signal to Alex that she did not wish him to open up in this way, and put a brake on the outpourings of his anxieties. However, she did not. Instead, having given prompts that she was encouraging him to go further, she now had to accept and work with what was being shared.

It may be, of course, that it is enough for Alex to have poured out his troubles and had a sympathetic, listening ear. However, Brenda is not even going to know that if she does not work with what has been presented.

Two factors will underpin her actions and how she responds to this encounter. The first is trust within the team that it is appropriate for Brenda to take on board and respond to the spiritual issues raised by a distressed patient. Secondly, issues of confidentiality should be explored within the team so that there is a clear understanding of what needs to be passed on and recorded, and what stays within the confines of the relationship between patient and professional.

Trust is vital and can only be developed if boundaries have been explored and understood. This requires that there is an acceptance within the team that everyone should be responsive to the deeper issues that might be raised, and not be deemed to be overstepping the mark if discussions move from the physical or practical to the spiritual or emotional. It is often only when physical distress is alleviated that a patient will feel comfortable with an exploration of other issues, including spiritual ones, which may have been masked or overwhelmed by pain or other physical problems.

There is a danger in the healthcare team that professionals become 'voyeurs', such that significant pieces of information are either shared in the spirit of 'I know something you don't know, and therefore the patient must trust me more than you' or 'I will not share this with you because I want to keep it to myself to preserve the privacy of the conversation.' There are issues which need to be shared, so that the whole team has an overview of a patient's circumstances, and there are issues which need not be, as they add little to an overall understanding of the patient's problems. These boundaries of confidentiality, and the decisions which arise from them about what is shared with the team, need to be explored and agreed upon. If there is no detailed discussion or existing protocols, these should be worked out on a case-by-case basis so that appropriate 'good practice' guidelines are established for the team.

Again, drawing on the continuation of Case Scenario 4.1, Reflective Activity 4.5 below enables you to broaden your understanding of your role in the healthcare team.

Reflective Activity 4.5

Continuing with our reflection on the continuing Case Scenario 4.1, if you were the healthcare professional in whom Alex has confided, how would you respond to the following questions:
- What issues might be raised by Alex that you would share with other team members?
- What issues might you keep in confidence and not share with the team?

One example of the need to be clear about professional boundaries might concern the issue of substance abuse. A patient may confide in you that they are a recovering alcoholic. They might do so to ensure that you understand some of the pressures they have experienced in earlier life, and to indicate some of the coping strategies they have developed. This would therefore be shared in the deepening of a pastoral relationship, and need not be shared in the wider team context. However, the patient's substance abuse may be ongoing. Consequently, with this knowledge, you may have a concern about potential access to alcohol and whether visitors might collude in its provision. As this may have a significant impact on social and/or medical issues for the patient, it is something of which the whole team should be aware.

REFERRAL CRITERIA

If we consider in Case Scenario 4.1 that Alex is in spiritual distress, this clearly cannot be ignored. If he has trusted a professional – and, by implication, the whole team in the healthcare environment – with his deeper feelings of fear, anxiety and concern, it is the responsibility of the professional concerned, in this case the physiotherapist, to take things further as appropriate. And it is important, therefore, for the team, and specific members within it, to look for suitable outcomes to alleviate Alex's distress.

All healthcare professionals can cite examples of missed communication – relevant information that was not passed on in a hand-over, assumptions being made that someone else will get to know the information, promises made to a patient that weren't kept because no action was taken, or scribbled notes being left that were never found. Such examples are commonplace. They are a result of a pressurised environment, busy professionals having too much to do, and pressing issues having to be responded to immediately so that the wider picture is compromised. There is no malice in this. Although there are of course examples of inadequate practice and lazy practitioners, on the whole healthcare professionals are not bad people, and they want the best for their patients.

So if on the one hand it is fundamental to the team that they are focused on the total well-being of a patient, including that patient's spiritual distress, and on the other hand examples of bad practice are not to become the norm, appropriate actions have to follow the revelation of distress, fear, anxiety and all that falls into the area of spiritual well-being.

Reflective Activity 4.6 will help you to develop your understanding of the teams in which you work and how you might initiate appropriate referrals.

Reflective Activity 4.6

Go back to the team members whom you identified in Reflective Activity 4.1, and taking the continuing case of Alex in Case Scenario 4.1 as an example, consider the following questions in relation to your own setting:
* Which members of the team would you expect to deal with Alex's issues?
* How would you initiate and word your referral?
* Would you consider referring to a chaplain? If so, why?

Although it is always appropriate to look within the healthcare team to facilitate referral and utilise the relevant skills of team members, there are times when the referral will go beyond the healthcare team in its widest sense. For example, there may be specific religious needs which are best met by a local faith or belief group representative who can be contacted by the chaplain. This should always be with the patient's consent and within agreed parameters of confidentiality. Cognisance should always be taken of what is recorded in the patient's clinical record. It may be necessary to have an agreed understanding of the language used, the appropriateness or otherwise of the issues recorded and the legal aspects of healthcare.

TEAM MEETINGS

Although it might not always be possible or practicable, all of the issues discussed above can be enhanced if the members of the healthcare team have regular opportunities to meet together. This, in an ideal setting, will not only be:

➤ to explore regularly the circumstances of the patient
➤ to get an update on what is happening, who is involved and what plans are being made with regard to the patient's care
➤ to ensure that decisions are appropriately recorded and members of the team are held accountable for agreed actions.

It will also be for the benefit of the team to meet together:

➤ to discuss working practices and how things might be improved, including tensions in the team (whether between individuals or relating to a specific case) that threaten to undermine the good working of the team
➤ to identify training needs and further development of protocols, procedures and the like
➤ to create an atmosphere of mutual support and respect.

Consequently, the healthcare team should have regular opportunities to meet together to explore all aspects of teamworking, both clinical and relational, in order to further develop good working practices and create and enhance a more satisfying working environment. Ultimately and most importantly, this will be of benefit to the holistic care that is offered to patients and their carers.

CHAPLAIN OR SPIRITUAL CARE PROFESSIONAL

In a large chaplaincy team, individual chaplaincy team members may be assigned as core members of specialist teams and units and also serve as members of the wider healthcare team in wards and departments. However, where the chaplain is a sole practitioner or in a small department they will have to prioritise their time and decide when and where they are a core or a wider member of the various healthcare teams. This skill of prioritising time in order to balance routine and emergency referrals and follow-up visits is recognised as a required competence by the UK Board of Healthcare Chaplaincy (1.1.7).[5]

This presupposes that there are systems in place for colleagues to make referrals to the chaplaincy department. Service standards for NHS Chaplaincy Services require all wards and departments to have a written protocol for referral to chaplaincy services readily available (2.5).[6]

An example of a referral protocol for specialist spiritual support is provided below. Reflective Activity 4.7 will guide you in examining its practicality and ease of use. You may want to compare it with what is in place in your own healthcare setting.

Procedure for referral for specialist spiritual support

Referral for specialist spiritual support will be to the chaplain once an assessment of spiritual and/or religious needs has been made. The chaplain, on engagement with the patient/carer, will further discern and assess the nature of the need and seek to meet that need or refer on to other internal or external resources as required.

1. Referral criteria

Patients/carers should be referred to the specialist chaplaincy service when one or more of the following applies:

➤ unmet spiritual needs have been assessed and acknowledged
➤ unmet religious needs have been assessed and acknowledged
➤ complex ethical issues have been identified and remain unresolved
➤ information is required regarding contact with other religious and spiritual care resources
➤ key concerns have been identified and are beyond the healthcare professional's competency to respond to
➤ conflict in individuals and families has been identified and remains unresolved
➤ emotional needs are unresolved and require further specialist assessment and intervention
➤ gaps in a healthcare professional's knowledge have been identified which require further explorations from a specialist, while not necessarily requiring the specialist to be directly engaged with the patient and/or carer.

2. Referral procedure

➤ Telephone the chaplaincy department and leave a message, including date and time.
➤ If it is an urgent referral, page the chaplain.
➤ Record the referral in the patient's notes, including date and time and details of referral.

Reflective Activity 4.7

From your own experience, evaluate the practicality of the above protocol by considering the following questions:
• Is this protocol workable?
• What are its strengths?
• Would you foresee any difficulties for those making referrals?

Simplicity and ease of use are strengths of any protocol. However, a protocol also has to be practical and effective.

Reflective Activity 4.8 will enable you to assess your own department's referral protocol for specialist spiritual care, evaluate its use, and consider ways in which it might be improved or made more effective.

Reflective Activity 4.8

Access your own chaplaincy department referral protocol and critically appraise its practicality and effectiveness.
- How would healthcare staff access the protocol? For example, where is it kept?
- How well does it work in practice?
- Is it effective in all clinical settings?
- How are new staff made aware of the protocol?
- In what ways could its use and availability be developed?

As patient throughput in hospital encourages shorter stays and increased numbers, chaplains are increasingly dependent on referrals from members of the healthcare team to fulfil their role and prioritise their time. Spiritual and religious assessment will be considered in more detail in Chapter 7. However, from this chapter we can conclude that commitment to effective working of the healthcare team is important, and clarification of the chaplain's role in that context is vital.

FURTHER READING

➤ McSherry W. *Making Sense of Spirituality in Nursing and Healthcare Practice: an integrated approach.* London: Jessica Kingsley Publishers; 2006.
➤ Royal College of Nursing. *RCN Survey on Spiritual Care in Nursing Practice.* www.rcn. org.uk/newsevents (accessed January 2010).

REFERENCES

1   Hearn J, Higginson I. Development and validation of a core outcome measure for palliative care: the palliative care outcome scale. *Quality in Health Care* 1999; **8:** 219–27.
2   Quality Improvement Scotland. *Standards for Integrated Care Pathways for Mental Health.* Edinburgh: Quality Improvement Scotland; 2007.
3   Clinical Standards Board for Scotland and the Scottish Partnership for Palliative Care. *Clinical Standards for Specialist Palliative Care.* Edinburgh: Clinical Standards Board for Scotland and the Scottish Partnership for Palliative Care; 2002.
4   Tebbit P. *Palliative Care 2000: commissioning through partnership.* London: National Council for Hospice and Specialist Palliative Care Services; 2000.
5   UK Board of Healthcare Chaplaincy. *Spiritual and Religious Care Capabilities and Competences for Healthcare Chaplains.* Cambridge: UK Board of Healthcare Chaplaincy; 2009.
6   UK Board of Healthcare Chaplaincy. *Standards for NHS Chaplaincy Services.* Cambridge: UK Board of Healthcare Chaplaincy; 2009.

CHAPTER 5

Competence in spiritual care

INTRODUCTION

Competences have been described as 'The complex synthesis of knowledge, skills, values, behaviours and attributes that enable individual professionals to work safely, effectively and legally within their particular scope of practice.'[1] Many healthcare professions are familiar with competences, and this might indicate that in all aspects of care, including a focus on spirituality, a simple understanding of competency will suffice. However, spiritual care as it is understood in the healthcare context is difficult to define, and does not lend itself to traditional measurement or analysis in its delivery. It is important, therefore, for healthcare professionals to find a balance between defining expectations in the delivery of spiritual care within a competency framework, and at the same time continuing to acknowledge the individuality of relationships between the patient/family/carer and professional in which important issues can be acknowledged and explored. Spiritual care should thus be seen as an 'art', and not just as a technical proficiency.

Consequently, the authors consider it to be more appropriate for the reader to engage in an exercise of self-assessment of their practice, rather than being offered a checklist of dos and don'ts, or a pro forma of how spiritual care can best be delivered. By exploring a framework for competence in spiritual care and examining practice through the preparation and analysis of a written reflective account of a significant event, the reader will be invited to engage in a process which will draw on their understanding and comprehension of the issues that have already been examined. Asking questions such as 'How self-aware am I?', 'How do I understand spirituality?', 'What is my role within the team in delivering spiritual care?' and 'How appropriate are my communication skills?' will allow the reader to build on their understanding of the aspects of spiritual care that were explored in the first four chapters of this book. In addition, it will encourage an examination of best practice. This will increase overall confidence in finding the necessary balance between defining competences and the discernment and individuality in the delivery of spiritual care.

WHAT IS COMPETENCY?

Before we proceed to elucidate the concept of competency, it is useful to consider an analogy from a non-healthcare setting. Suppose that we decide to do away with our coal fire and replace it with a new gas appliance. We buy the fire from an appropriate store, and choose the one which is suitable for our own needs. However, most of us cannot install such an appliance ourselves, and the law prohibits us from doing so. Therefore, we look around for someone who has the skills, knowledge and experience to do this for us. There are many such people who offer their services in the 'small ads' of our local paper. But how do we know which one to choose? There may be recommendations from individuals who have used such tradespeople before. But how do we know which gas fitters are bona fide and which ones might be 'cowboys'? We choose the ones who are properly registered because we know that according to safety and legal standards they are the only ones who are competent and who can be designated as 'qualified'. We shall then know that our gas fire will be fitted safely and that we have some recourse if the work is not carried out to the agreed level of competency.

The same is true for all healthcare professions. When any professional in a healthcare setting is expected to work within a system of agreed competence or to a set of defined professional standards, a clearly understood framework can be developed against which effectiveness and fitness to practise can be assessed, measured and developed.

COMPETENCY AND INDIVIDUALITY

No matter how important competence is, individuality in the delivery of spiritual care continues to be crucial. 'When a person is treated with respect, when they are listened to in a meaningful way, when they are seen and treated as a whole person within the context of their life, values and beliefs, then they are receiving spiritual care.'[2] Consequently, we need to retain the importance of the 'freedom to be' and the uniqueness of our relationship with the service user in any investigation of competence.

In 2003, a multi-disciplinary group of healthcare professionals within the Marie Curie Cancer Care organisation worked on definitions of competency in the delivery of spiritual and religious care.[3] The framework was developed for use in specialist palliative care, and was recommended by the National Institute for Clinical Excellence and adopted by the Association of Hospice and Palliative Care Chaplains as their working framework.[4] The framework has also proved to be readily adaptable to all healthcare settings. It has been utilised as a resource for further developments within the NHS and, in particular, within healthcare chaplaincy professional organisations.[5-7]

The Marie Curie Cancer Care competency framework defines four levels of engagement with service users in the delivery of spiritual and religious care. As can be seen from the following extract, the levels are correlated with the professional responsibility for members of staff and their contact with patients and their carers:[8]

> **Level 1:** All staff and volunteers who have casual contact with their patients and their families. This level seeks to ensure that all staff and volunteers understand that all people have spiritual needs, and distinguishes between spiritual and religious needs. It seeks to encourage basic skills of awareness, relationships and communication, and an ability to refer concerns to members of the multi-disciplinary team (MDT).
>
> **Level 2:** All staff and volunteers whose duties require contact with patients and families/carers. This level seeks to enhance the competences developed at level 1 with an increased awareness of spiritual and religious needs and how they might be identified and responded to. In addition to increased communication skills, identification and referral of difficult needs should be achievable along with an ability to identify personal training needs.
>
> **Level 3:** Staff and volunteers who are members of the MDT. This level seeks to further enhance the skills of levels 1 and 2. It moves into the area of assessment of spiritual and religious need, developing a plan for care and recognising complex spiritual, religious and ethical issues. This level also introduces confidentiality and the recording of sensitive and personal patient information.
>
> **Level 4:** Staff and volunteers whose primary responsibility is for the spiritual and religious care of patients, visitors and staff. Staff working at this level are expected to be able to manage and facilitate complex spiritual and religious needs in patients, families/carers, staff and volunteers. In particular, they will deal with the existential and practical needs arising from the impact on individuals and families from illness, life, dying and death. In addition, they should have a clear understanding of their own personal beliefs and be able to journey with others focused on other people's needs and agenda. They should liaise with external resources as required. They should also act as a resource for support, training and education of healthcare professionals and volunteers, and seek to be involved in professional and national initiatives.

In adapting this framework for use in the wider healthcare setting, the term 'multi-disciplinary team' should be understood in terms of the core healthcare team as outlined in Chapter 4. There is an expectation that all allied health professionals, doctors and nurses would be working at level 3.

SELF-ASSESSMENT

Understanding the expectations and implications of working at an agreed level of competency in the delivery of spiritual care can be useful. This will not only create an ability to assess both performance and outcomes, but will also allow the practitioner to identify areas of education and development necessary to allow them to properly fulfil their role.

Level 3 of the competence framework indicates that this level – at which all members of the core healthcare team are expected to operate – carries with it the expectation that the basics of knowledge, skills and appropriate actions in relation to spiritual care are fundamental. However, this level seeks to enhance these basics by moving into the assessment of spiritual and religious need, development of an appropriate plan of care, recognising complex spiritual, religious and ethical issues and when to refer on. It also introduces confidentiality and the recording of sensitive and personal patient information.

This process of development is summarised in Table 5.1.[9]

Table 5.1

Competences		
Knowledge	*Skills*	*Actions*
In addition to the knowledge at levels 1 and 2, everyone working at level 3 should be able to: <ul><li>Understand the nature of spiritual assessment, including the religious and ethical dimensions</li><li>Understand the skills that other members of the MDT possess in relation to spiritual care</li><li>Understand confidentiality with regard to patients' and carers' personal information and what may be shared within the MDT</li></ul>	In addition to the skills at levels 1 and 2, everyone working at level 3 should have the following skills: <ul><li>An ability to describe and evidence a working definition of spiritual and religious needs</li><li>An ability to elicit patients' key concerns at a pace directed by patients</li><li>An ability to recognise unmet spiritual and religious need</li><li>An ability to recognise and respond appropriately to conflict in individuals and families and to emotional issues</li><li>An ability to develop and administer a plan for spiritual care based on spiritual or religious need</li><li>An ability to recognise complex spiritual, religious and ethical issues</li><li>An ability to refer effectively to other spiritual care resources, including chaplaincy, and to clearly articulate reasons for referral</li><li>An ability to identify education, training and development needs</li><li>An ability to respect confidentiality and the appropriate disclosure of patient/carer personal information</li></ul>	In addition to the performance at levels 1 and 2, everyone working at level 3 should be able to demonstrate an ability to: <ul><li>Document patient/carer information in a way that respects confidentiality of individuals and of the MDT</li><li>Document the assessment, interventions (care) and outcomes for patients and carers</li><li>Document appropriate referrals following spiritual assessment (e.g. referral to chaplaincy or the patient's own faith representative)</li></ul>

It is essential, therefore, with such importance given to the engagement with spiritual issues, that the healthcare professional should be able to reflect on, analyse and assess their practice. This can be done through a review of documentation – that is, asking whether the documentation demonstrates spiritual assessment, shows an understanding of a respect for confidentiality, details interventions, reveals appropriate care planning and outcomes, and indicates referral when appropriate. However, as we have indicated above, this can easily lend itself to a 'tick-box' process whereby competence is measured only by definable actions and outcomes. If the balance is to be right, a review of practice should be integral to any Personal Performance Review and Development (PPRD) process or appraisal system, so that practice is explored, issues are examined and training needs are identified.

Integral to such an approach is the preparation of a written reflective account of a significant event or case review. The self-assessment process in the following Reflective Activities therefore forms the core of this chapter.

Reflective Activity 5.1

Consider a significant event in which you were involved. As guidance, the following will be useful to your thought processes.
- Reflect on the important aspects of the event which relate to the spiritual, religious or ethical needs of the patient or their family members.
- Recall the 'when' and the 'how' of the eliciting of key concerns, and consider whether this was at an appropriate pace as determined by the service user.
- Ask yourself whether unmet spiritual and/or religious needs were identified.
- Consider how and when a plan of action/care evolved, if at all.
- Remind yourself of resources, either within yourself or external to the event, which were drawn upon.
- Reflect on your confidence in dealing with, assessing and taking forward the issues that were raised in this event.
- Consider the effect that this had on you, and what you did with that.
- Reflect on the outcome for, and benefit to, the service user.

Guided by these points, write a reflective account of this significant event that might be used as a self-assessment account or utilised in a PPRD process.

An example of a written reflective account can be found in Chapter 12, Case Scenario 12.2. When you have completed your written reflective account, Reflective Activity 5.2 will enable you to complete a self-assessment of your competence.

Reflective Activity 5.2

From your written reflective account, complete the following self-assessment which has been adapted from the Marie Curie Cancer Care self-assessment tool.[10] Remember, though, that not all accounts will enable you to evidence all competences and some may be unmet for that reason.

Knowledge	Met	Unmet
Awareness of own spirituality		
Understand the importance and impact of verbal and non-verbal communication		
Understand the nature of spiritual assessment		
Understand the skills other members of the team have in relation to spiritual care		
Understand confidentiality and what might/should be shared with other members of the multi-disciplinary team (MDT)		

Skills	Met	Unmet
An ability to develop a rapport with the service user		
A recognition of my own personal limitations		
An ability to listen actively and demonstrate empathy		
An ability to recognise and respond appropriately to emotions expressed		
A recognition of my own limitations in managing difficult issues		
Appropriate referral to other members of the MDT		
An ability to describe and evidence a working definition of spiritual and religious needs		
An ability to elicit key concerns at a pace determined by the service user		
An ability to recognise and respond appropriately to emotional and conflict issues		
An ability to develop and administer an appropriate plan of care		
An ability to recognise complex issues		
An ability to refer effectively to other spiritual care resources, including chaplaincy, and clearly articulate reasons for referral		
An ability to identify training needs which this scenario has highlighted		
An ability to respect confidentiality and appropriate disclosure of service-user information		

(continued)

Action	Met	Unmet
Appropriate relationships with patients and their families were built		
Supportive listening was provided for the patient and/or carer		
Patient/carer information was documented in a way that respected the confidentiality of individuals and the MDT		
Assessment, interventions and outcomes were appropriately documented		
Referrals following a spiritual assessment were documented appropriately, including referrals to chaplaincy or the service user's own faith representative		

To complete the self-assessment process, Reflective Activity 5.3 will enable you to review those areas of competence that are unmet, and to identify issues for professional development and training.

Reflective Activity 5.3

Having reviewed the 'met' and 'unmet' issues in the grid prepared in Reflective Activity 5.2, consider the following questions:
- What areas of spiritual care are you particularly confident in?
- What areas of spiritual care would you identify as needing work?
- What issues does this raise for your practice?
- What training needs have been identified?
- What personal issues has this raised for you?

To further develop your personal competence you could consider taking this self-assessment for discussion at your next clinical supervision or appraisal session. This exercise could also be adapted and used as a training resource by senior staff to encourage spiritual competence in other team members.

Having identified the knowledge, skills and actions necessary for appropriate functioning at any level of competency, it is important for the healthcare setting to have systems in place to enhance the quality of care offered. Developing competence in spiritual care enables the blending of skills, knowledge and action with the processes of intuitive and individual response to spiritual and religious need. A working knowledge of competency levels, an understanding of the limitations and boundaries at each level, and an awareness of referral options to a higher level of competency, when appropriate, are all essential. This enables best and safe practice in spiritual care.

CHAPLAIN OR SPIRITUAL CARE LEAD

In a healthcare culture in which competences are both familiar and well utilised for a range of healthcare professions, the logical progression leads to the production of a definable competency framework for healthcare chaplains. Such a framework can help chaplains to articulate what spiritual and religious care is and how it can be assessed and provided. A framework can also identify the complexities of spiritual and religious care and the expertise of those who are appointed to assess and address such needs. Finally, a competency framework can be used by educationalists to develop professional education for those seeking to enter the profession and those seeking to develop their expertise. Such a framework was developed and published by NHS Scotland, and has been adopted for use throughout the UK by the UK Board of Healthcare Chaplaincy.[11,12]

Capabilities and competences

The Departments of Health and professional organisations in the UK use different terminology that is sometimes confused. The words 'capability' and 'competence' can be used synonymously. However, the Spiritual and Religious Care Capabilities and Competences for Healthcare Chaplains clearly distinguish between the terms, and believe that both are essential.

The distinction between the terms 'competence' and 'capability' can be described as follows:[13]

➤ **Competence** describes what individuals know or are able to do in terms of knowledge, skills and attitudes at a particular point in time.

➤ **Capability** describes the extent to which an individual can apply, adapt and synthesise new knowledge from experience and continue to improve his or her performance.

It has also been suggested that competences do not take into account complexity, and that effective practitioners need more than a prescribed set of competences to carry out their roles effectively.[14,15] The authors affirm that the chaplain is the point of referral for the complexities of spiritual care. It follows, therefore, that if the chaplaincy service is to be assessed against clear standards of professional performance as it responds to such complexities, it is necessary for chaplains, and others, to be aware of the capabilities and competences that they are expected to have for the effective delivery of that service.

CAPABILITIES AND COMPETENCES FRAMEWORK

NHS Education for Scotland and the UK Board of Healthcare Chaplaincy, in their Spiritual and Religious Care Capabilities and Competences for Healthcare Chaplains, have created a framework that enables chaplains to evidence competence and demonstrate capability through a process of continuing professional development. In so doing, they offered the following *raison d'être*:

> ... the logical progression is to produce a capability and competence framework for individuals working as healthcare chaplains. This framework would help to inform and develop education and training, the planning of work-based learning and of personal development of healthcare chaplains. The document is referenced to the Chaplaincy Standards and linked to the Knowledge and Skills Framework.[16]

Healthcare chaplains are expected to demonstrate the ability to adapt to frequent change and complex situations. This ability incorporates professional judgement, decision-making skills and experiential knowledge gained from many situations. Consequently, the capability framework for chaplains focuses on areas which, in their totality, encapsulate all that is expected of chaplains, namely:[17]

➤ realising people's full potential
➤ developing the ability to adapt and apply knowledge and skills
➤ learning from experience
➤ envisaging the future and contributing to making it happen.

Structure of the framework

The Capabilities Framework for Healthcare Chaplains is presented under four domains, each of which contains a number of detailed elements.

➤ **Knowledge and skills for professional practice**, including: knowledge and skills needed to practise effectively; an understanding of good ethical practice; communication skills; appropriate education and training.
➤ **Spiritual and religious assessment and intervention**, including: an understanding of both spiritual and religious assessment issues and intervention opportunities, and the distinction between the two.
➤ **Institutional practice**, including: teamworking; staff support; issues of chaplaincy to the hospital or unit.
➤ **Reflective practice**, including: the importance of reflective practice for optimum performance; explorations of personal spiritual development.

The following case scenario and reflective activities will enable you to tease out what working in these four domains might mean in your practice.

CASE SCENARIO 5.1

Terry is 63 years old, and has been admitted to the ward during a major depressive episode. His next of kin is recorded as his wife, Alison, and she is a regular visitor to the ward. She and Terry have no other family. Alison indicates that she does not wish any information about Terry's care and circumstances to be given to anyone else. Appropriate medication has been

(continued)

prescribed, and Terry is on the ward for several weeks. During a care procedure, when no one else is present, Terry confides to you that there is another woman in his life. He says that he has been living a 'double life' for a number of years and that his 'other partner' is the most important person in his life at the present time. He states that his marriage is 'a sham', and he would very much like his partner, Mary, to be allowed to come and visit him, so long as his wife doesn't get to know about this. Terry states that this situation has been 'getting him down' and he feels that he needs to 'do something about it'. He has never confided in anyone else, and asks for your help 'to work it out'.

Reflective Activity 5.4

From your own experience, and recalling the self-assessment process undertaken in Reflective Activities 5.1, 5.2 and 5.3, consider the following questions in relation to Case Scenario 5.1.
- Would you consider Terry's needs to be spiritual?
- Is there a need for Terry's circumstances to be referred on to you as a specialist?
- What might be offered by way of a therapeutic response?
- What might you expect the outcome of this scenario to be?

Spiritual care, including discernment of spiritual needs and assessment of the delivery of appropriate care, is not easy. It requires constant sensitivity and self-awareness if the needs of a patient like Terry are to be met. Reflective Activity 5.5 will help us explore this further.

Reflective Activity 5.5

Returning to Case Scenario 5.1:
- What implications does Terry's request for his 'other partner' to visit raise for you professionally? For example, what are the implications with regard to:
  - visiting arrangements?
  - next of kin?
- What issues does Terry's request for his 'other partner' to visit raise for you as an individual? For example, what are the issues with regard to your personal feelings?
- What might be the knowledge, skills and abilities necessary for you as a chaplain to offer effective care to Terry?

It may be that you identify your need to be up to date with your knowledge of current thinking and research into aspects of spiritual and religious care, so that you use this in understanding Terry's issues and offering an effective response. There may be ethical issues here, too, including a potential 'clash' between your own moral stance and what is best for Terry. Your communication skills will also be important here.

Reflective Activity 5.6

Continuing to reflect on Case Scenario 5.1:
- What assessment might you make of Terry's needs?
- What interventions might you formulate to respond to those needs?

It may be that you are able to clarify matters, in partnership with Terry, in the immediacy of your engagement with him. However, it may be necessary to reflect personally on the issues after the encounter is over, or to share that exploration of assessment and intervention issues with the wider team. In either case, you will be considering what resources might be available to Terry and/ or his family, from yourself or the team setting, always being aware of referral options to other internal or external care providers.

Reflective Activity 5.7

Continuing to reflect on Case Scenario 5.1:
- What are the implications of this scenario for the wider healthcare team?
- How would you communicate this encounter within the team?
- What would you record in the patient notes?

Issues which arise here concern the chaplain's role in the immediacy of a team setting or in the wider healthcare context, as well as in relationships with other healthcare professionals. It may be that reference needs to be made to agreed protocols or procedures. In addition, working relationships will play a part, as will issues of confidentiality, the giving and receiving of ongoing support, and the personalities of the individuals involved.

The final reflective activity will enable you to consider how as chaplains we might process such complex scenarios and the processes and dilemmas that have been worked through in the previous reflective activities.

Reflective Activity 5.8

Reflecting on the implications from Case Scenario 5.1 that have been explored above:
- What might be the issues which you, as a chaplain, could constructively reflect on? For example:
  - the ethical and moral conflicts in the scenario
  - your personal feelings and beliefs
  - your role as a member of the healthcare team
  - confidentiality and the documenting of your encounter and any intervention.

If this was a real scenario that you were reflecting on:
- How might you use this reflection in your professional development? For example:
  - discuss it with your clinical or pastoral supervisor
  - discuss it with colleagues

(continued)

> – present the issues as complex case review for the healthcare team
> – develop the case as a journal article.

Reference to the Spiritual and Religious Care Capabilities and Competences for Healthcare Chaplains makes it clear that the chaplaincy role is held and offered in a professional and evidential context. The chaplain is expected to operate at the highest level of ability in the delivery of spiritual care. It emphasises the need for a fully equipped, appropriately competent, experienced, trained and accountable professional. Such a practitioner acts with, and on behalf of, the whole healthcare team to ensure that the most complex issues, as well as aspects which arise in the breadth of spiritual care at all levels, are appropriately and effectively responded to.

The expectation is that chaplains will have the confidence of the healthcare professionals who together form the healthcare team. If this is to be borne out in practice, those who refer or seek support to meet the often complex needs of individuals who require spiritual and religious care have to be assured of the competence of the spiritual care lead. Chaplains should therefore be able to demonstrate that they are capable and competent practitioners.

FURTHER READING

➤ Baldacchino D. Nursing competencies for spiritual care. *Journal of Clinical Nursing* 2006; **15**: 885–96.

➤ Gordon T, Mitchell D. A competency model for the assessment and delivery of spiritual care. *Palliative Medicine* 2004; **18**: 646–51.

➤ Kerry M. Towards competence: a narrative and framework for spiritual caregivers. In: Orchard H (ed.) *Spirituality in Health Care Contexts*. London: Jessica Kingsley Publishers; 2001. pp. 118–32.

➤ Skills for Health. *Competences*. http://skillsforhealth.org.uk/competences.aspx (accessed December 2010).

➤ Talbot M. Monkey see, monkey do: a critique of the competency model in graduate education. *Medical Education* 2004; **38**: 580–1.

➤ van Leeuwen R, Cusveller B. Nursing competencies for spiritual care. *Journal of Advanced Nursing* 2004; **48**: 234–46.

➤ van Leeuwen R, Tiesings L, Middel B *et al.* The validity and reliability of an instrument to assess nursing competencies spiritual care. *Journal of Clinical Nursing* 2009; **18**: 2857–69.

REFERENCES

1 Roberts S. Continuing professional development: what the future might hold. *Journal of Sports Medicine* 2004; **19**: 14–16.

2 NHS Education for Scotland. *Spiritual and Religious Care Capabilities and Competences for Healthcare Chaplains*. Edinburgh: NHS Education for Scotland; 2008.

3 Marie Curie Cancer Care. *Spiritual and Religious Care Competencies for Specialist Palliative Care*. London: Marie Curie Cancer Care; 2003.

4 National Institute for Clinical Excellence. *Improving Supportive and Palliative Care for Adults with Cancer. Manual*. London: National Institute for Clinical Excellence; 2004.

5 Welsh Assembly Government. *Guidance on Capabilities and Competences for Healthcare Chaplains/Spiritual Care Givers in Wales*. Cardiff: Welsh Assembly Government; 2010. www.cymru.gov.uk (accessed November 2010).

6 UK Board of Healthcare Chaplaincy. *Spiritual and Religious Care Capabilities and Competences for Healthcare Chaplains*. Cambridge: UK Board of Healthcare Chaplaincy; 2009.

7 NHS Education for Scotland. *Spiritual and Religious Care Capabilities and Competences for Healthcare Chaplains*, op. cit.

8 Marie Curie Cancer Care. *Spiritual and Religious Care Competencies for Specialist Palliative Care*, op. cit.

9 Marie Curie Cancer Care. *Spiritual and Religious Care Competencies for Specialist Palliative Care*, op. cit., p. 5.

10 Marie Curie Cancer Care. *Spiritual and Religious Care Competencies for Specialist Palliative Care: assessment tools and self-assessment tools*. London: Marie Curie Cancer Care; 2004.

11 Marie Curie Cancer Care. *Spiritual and Religious Care Competencies for Specialist Palliative Care*, op. cit.

12 UK Board of Healthcare Chaplaincy. *Spiritual and Religious Care Capabilities and Competences for Healthcare Chaplains*, op. cit.

13 Fraser SW, Greenhalgh T. Coping with complexity: educating for capability. *British Medical Journal* 2001; **323**: 799–803.

14 Wilson T, Holt T. Complexity and clinical care. *British Medical Journal* 2001; **323**: 685–8.

15 Sainsbury Centre for Mental Health. *The Capable Practitioner*. London: Sainsbury Centre for Mental Health; 2001.

16 Department of Health. *The NHS Knowledge and Skills Framework (NHS KSF) and the Development Review Process*. London: Department of Health; 2004.

17 UK Board of Healthcare Chaplaincy. *Spiritual and Religious Care Capabilities and Competences for Healthcare Chaplains*, op. cit.

CHAPTER 6

Disentangling spiritual and religious care

INTRODUCTION

The relationship between spiritual and religious care is complex. It is significantly influenced by the cultural (societal and familial) context, experience, beliefs and values of those who seek to describe it. For many in Western society, especially in the USA, the two words are often used synonymously. However, increasingly in healthcare in many European countries the term 'spiritual' is understood to be a broader concept which includes, but is not confined to, what has been traditionally referred to as 'religious.'

Increasingly, service users and healthcare staff are not actively involved in faith communities. However, some may still perceive the church, synagogue or mosque that they attended as a child as their spiritual home, and hold dear some fundamentals of the beliefs and moral teaching which they absorbed at home or in places of worship in their formative years. Religious beliefs and values may still influence many people's worldviews and decision making, but if they are not regular worshippers they often would not consider themselves religious. Nor would many, if asked, be definite about describing themselves as 'spiritual', as this is a term which although increasingly in use still has vague 'New Age', alternative-lifestyle or non-conformist connotations. Spirituality as a concept is very difficult to define. Indeed, it can be argued that by seeking to create a clear definition of spirituality something is immediately lost – mystery, otherness and subjectivity being intrinsic to whatever spirituality might be (*see* also Chapter 1 for reflective activities which will help you to explore your own understanding of what spirituality means). Reflective Activity 6.1 will allow you to explore religious and spiritual associations.

Reflective Activity 6.1

With what are the terms 'spiritual' and 'religious' associated for you?

Create two columns, one with the heading 'Spiritual' and the other with the heading 'Religion/religious.'

Now brainstorm all of the ideas, feelings, images, experiences and descriptions that come to mind which you associate with these terms, under each heading.

Spiritual	*Religion/religious*

After you have created a full list for both, mark each entry, where appropriate, with a plus or minus sign to depict whether each association is positive or negative. If a particularly vivid connection is made or a strong feeling is evoked then mark it twice. Leave a blank if a more neutral response is felt.

RELIGION AND SPIRITUALITY: SUBJECTIVE UNDERSTANDINGS

As engagement with Reflective Activity 6.1 may have revealed, the consideration of religious and spiritual issues is an emotive subject, often evoking strong opinion as well as feeling. This exercise is an important one. Not only may it reveal the depth and range of emotions and experiences, both positive and negative, that any healthcare worker may have in relation to religion and spirituality, but also it gives you a glimpse of how you may inwardly react to spiritual and religious issues that may arise in clinical encounters with particular service users. The inner responses that are experienced in relation to others significantly inform a practitioner's ability to relate meaningfully with another, for good or ill, especially if the practitioner is unaware of the origin of strongly felt emotions or reactions to another's story. If we have some degree of awareness of what we bring as part of our story with regard to religion and spirituality and to relationships with others, then we will be better able to separate out service users' feelings, understandings and opinions from our own. This will allow us to concentrate more fully on their spiritual and religious concerns, while any perturbing or strong reactions within us can be noted, shelved, and then addressed at a later date with a trusted other.

In Chapter 1 you were encouraged to explore your spirituality. Reflective Activities 6.2 and 6.3 will help you to unravel what religion might mean for you and those you care for in both your personal and professional life.

Reflective Activity 6.2

To develop an awareness of what place and role religion has in your *personal* life, in the past or present, reflect on the following questions:
- To what extent has religion had a role in your formation and development as a person?
  - For example, to what extent has it influenced who you are, what you believe and how you make decisions in life?
- Think about your exposure to religious beliefs and practices when you were growing up, both at home and at school, including the influence of relations or friends.
  - For example, what has your involvement been in any religious services or practices, whether this was regular or occasional (e.g. attending funerals, weddings, a bar mitzvah, Christmas or Easter services)?
- Has faith or belief played a part in how you have dealt with personal losses or times of adversity?
- Have you participated in any rituals in relation to national or global tragedies, such as 9/11?
- To what extent has the place of religion in your life changed since you were at school?

Reflective Activity 6.3

To develop an awareness of what place and role religion has in your *professional* life, follow the steps below:
- Make a list of ways in which you have observed patients or their carers being positively comforted, supported or encouraged by their faith, its practice and membership of their faith community.
- Now reflect on any experiences you have had with service users when their religious beliefs or practices or membership of a faith community caused or added to their distress.
- To what extent has your experience as a healthcare practitioner changed your understanding of religion?
- To these lists add your reflections on how religious belief, practices and faith communities are of benefit to local and global communities.
- Now note how you have observed religious belief, practices and faith communities being less than helpful to individual and community well-being, both locally and globally.
- Finally, read over your responses to the above and summarise what you perceive religion to be and its significance in healthcare.

The authors believe that a subjective or personal awareness of what spirituality and religion mean to each practitioner is of paramount importance for the delivery of competent and sensitive spiritual and religious care. However, in order to further the exploration of the relationship between spiritual and religious care, a couple of objective descriptions are offered.

HOW RELIGION AND SPIRITUALITY ARE RELATED: OBJECTIVE DESCRIPTIONS

The Scottish Government has provided one approach to conceptualising the relationship between spiritual and religious care delivered in a healthcare setting:[1]

> **Spiritual care** is usually given in a one-to-one relationship, is completely person-centred, and makes no assumption about personal conviction or life orientation.

> **Religious care** is given in the context of shared religious beliefs, values, liturgies and lifestyle of a faith community.

> Spiritual care is not necessarily religious. Religious care should always be spiritual.

> Spiritual care might be said to be the umbrella term of which religious care is a part. It is the intention of religious care to meet spiritual need.

Stephen Wright's description of the relationship is also helpful:[2]

> Everybody is spiritual, but not everyone is religious. We all seek meaning, purpose, relationship and connectedness in life, but not everybody chooses to channel that quest through the more formal structure and belief system of a religion.

SPIRITUAL CARE IS BROADER THAN RELIGIOUS CARE

Not all of the spiritual needs of a religious patient or carer will be met when healthcare practitioners facilitate the provision of appropriate religious care. Meaning and purpose, comfort and hope may be found by bringing to mind certain beliefs, reading sacred texts, or through prayer and sharing in relevant rituals. Enabling patients to access quiet spaces and perform any necessary ablutions before praying or contacting the healthcare chaplain or a representative of the patient's faith community may have a significant role in meeting, in part, their spiritual needs. However, all religious people will also have relationships, activities and connections other than faith-related ones, which make their life worth living. To meet a person's religious needs is only to meet *some* of their spiritual needs. In addition, it is all too easy to assume that the most important spiritual need of a religious patient or a carer at any one time is to utilise the resources (inner or outer) that their faith affords them. During a patient's journey of dealing with illness, injury, accident or impending death, their most significant and immediate spiritual need will change with time according to their circumstance, mood, and level of awareness of their prognosis. Sometimes it will take the form of a religious need, but often it will not. To ensure best and person-centred practice, healthcare staff need to *ask the patient or carer* what is most important to them in the 'here and now.' If it is a spiritual issue, how can the healthcare team help them to meet that need?

Case Scenario 6.1 will probe what it means for us to see beyond immediate assumptions.

CASE SCENARIO 6.1

Jean was a devout Roman Catholic who, when she was well enough, attended Mass every morning at her local chapel. However, due to a worsening of her chronic obstructive airways disease she became more confined to her home, with increasingly regular admissions to the local hospital due to chest infections and/or severe breathlessness. Jean's local parish priest and lay visitors were regular callers at her home and the Roman Catholic hospital chaplain and his visiting team were similarly attentive in the hospital, ensuring that her religious-ritual needs were regularly met. Jean appreciated all of this but during a particularly lengthy stay in hospital she became low in mood and more withdrawn than usual. One of the staff nurses on the ward became acutely aware of Jean's melancholia one afternoon and automatically asked her if she would like to see the chaplain. Jean didn't take the nurse up on the offer, which surprised the staff. Later, when there was a lull in ward activity, the same nurse returned to sit beside Jean and to find out what was going on for her that day. She gently explored what was important to Jean in her life apart from her faith and how she had coped with difficult times in the past. Jean, hesitantly at first, began to talk about her garden and how she loved to spend time in it, especially tending her flowers. Her garden was Jean's oasis in life, a place of tranquillity, where she quite literally 'smelt the roses'. The nurse asked Jean if she would like to go outside to enjoy the rose garden in the hospital grounds that evening. Weather permitting, every visiting time after that during Jean's stay her friends and relatives wheeled her in a wheelchair, with oxygen cylinder and nasal cannula and all, to the rose garden. Jean's spirits lifted and when she got home the pattern continued. Several months later, on Jean's final admission to hospital, she was bed-ridden – so the flowers from the hospital grounds and her garden came to her in a vase.

Jean's spiritual needs were met only in part by meeting her religious needs. Further enquiry allowed her spiritual needs to be more fully met.

RELIGIOUS AND SPIRITUAL CARE: ASK THE PATIENT

In seeking to provide person-centred and timely spiritual and religious care, the authors believe that objective definitions or descriptions, although they are helpful pointers, are of secondary importance to asking service users what they actually need and how healthcare practitioners can help to meet those needs. When assessing patients' spiritual needs, healthcare staff have to begin at the point where patients and carers actually are in their particular journey through life in relation to spiritual and religious matters, not at the point where it is assumed that they are. Many patients will not want their spiritual needs to be met through religious practices, even though they have a particular religious label entered on a hospital admission form. For many people from a variety of ethnic and social groupings, stating their religious affiliation is perhaps more a cultural expression of their identity than an expression of faith or belief. For example, a patient who describes him- or herself as Jewish or Muslim may belong to a family that has been non-practising for one or two generations. Similarly, for a patient who states that they are Protestant on admission to a hospital in the west of Scotland, this may be more about articulating that they are not Roman Catholic than about stating that they are a practising Presbyterian.

In some areas of the UK, such as large parts of Scotland and Northern Ireland, the ethnic population is small and the numbers of service users who come from faith groups outside the main Christian denominations are low. It can be anxiety-provoking for members of healthcare staff, as well as for patients, when someone from a minority faith is admitted into their care. We want to provide the best possible holistic care, including meeting the patient's spiritual and cultural needs, but have little exposure to working with minority groups. Sometimes there is a tendency immediately to take the multi-faith handbook from the wardroom shelf or to search the Internet to find out what needs a patient of a different creed, colour or culture may have. This is to be commended, and there are certainly some helpful resources available if these are required. However, it is important to avoid making assumptions. As a first step, take time to ask and learn from the patients and carers themselves. They are the real experts.

Case Scenario 6.2 emphasises the importance of asking the patient.

CASE SCENARIO 6.2

Samina is a 30-year-old married Scottish university lecturer who, when asked on admission to her local hospice, stated that her religion was Muslim. Her husband, Mo, is a PhD student, originally from Somalia, who came to Scotland to study. Mo was also brought up as a Muslim, but neither he nor Samina are actively involved in their local faith community. However, they are both highly respectful of their parents' beliefs, and hold dearly the values that they absorbed as children within their family homes. They have only been married for 18 months.

On passing the hospice quiet room one day shortly after Samina's admission, you see Mo with his head in his hands looking distraught. You approach him and ask gently whether he wants some company. He replies 'Samina says it's Allah's will that she is dying. She wants me to get on with my life, to visit less and get on with my studies and finish my PhD this year.' He sobs, and then after a while he says 'I can't. I want to be here as much as I am able.'

From your reading of Case Scenario 6.2, consider your responses to the questions in Reflective Activity 6.4 below.

Reflective Activity 6.4

- What are the issues that may be involved in Case Scenario 6.2?
- How would you respond?
- How best can you help both Mo and Samina?

CASE SCENARIO 6.2 CONTINUED

Several days later it is clear that Samina is now dying. She has openly talked with Mo and her brother and sister, Hafis and Mona, about what her wishes are regarding her funeral. She does not want to upset her parents, but she does not want all of the traditional rituals that are performed in the Muslim community around a time of death.

You meet Samina's parents in the corridor shortly after you hear about the situation from the chaplain at the multi-disciplinary meeting. Samina's mother begins to cry, and Samina's father begins to talk in a raised voice about Mo's lack of respect and the family making decisions contrary to the way they were brought up.

Reflective Activity 6.5

Now, as Case Scenario 6.2 unfolds, reflect on the following questions:
- How would you respond?
- What issues may be important for the different individuals involved?
- How best can you help the whole family?

The key here is to ask the patient or the family member or carer with whom you are involved what their needs are. You will not have all of the necessary information and knowledge at your fingertips, which is all the more reason why you should draw on information which those with whom you are working can be encouraged to share.

HELPLESSNESS AS PART OF OUR HUMANITY

Whatever the natural abilities or limitations of any healthcare practitioner, and whatever capabilities and competences are learned and developed, the authors believe that one of the greatest challenges that is faced when delivering holistic care is that there are always things that we cannot fix. In caring for others there will be tensions that cannot be relieved, needs that go unmet, and pain for which there is no soothing balm. This is hard. Feeling helpless and useless in the face of great suffering is difficult to live with, especially in a healthcare system that is still task-oriented and values 'doing' more than 'being with', and that values curing more than alleviating and caring. In such a culture, to experience such helplessness may feel like failure. However, it is far from it – to feel this way is to be human. Paradoxically and profoundly, to be human is to be most professional and proficient in providing spiritual care. This will be explored more fully in Chapter 8.

For a healthcare professional to recognise and own personal helplessness in challenging and messy situations is far from being a weakness. Indeed, it may be a point of contact with the lived experience of the patient and/or carers involved. At such moments, the feeling of the practitioner may echo something of the feelings of the patient and carers. If healthcare professionals are able to stay with their helplessness in difficult, irresolvable situations and remain with patients and carers, where appropriate, as they experience helplessness and even hopelessness, these professionals may truly be a comforting, hopeful and memorable presence. Ironically, it is sometimes when practitioners feel most helpless and useless, and the struggle to remain steadfastly with others is greatest, that patients and families are most grateful. Being brave is not about living without fear and uncertainty. Quite the opposite – it is about functioning and still caring despite the helplessness and uncertainty that are felt. Real courage involves being able to admit to oneself and to others, at times, that none of us have all the answers. It involves saying 'I don't know' and still being available. This is spiritual care, not religious care, which is of great value because it utilises the human gifts of love, compassion, real courage and discernment which not everyone possesses to the same degree.

The complexities of supporting others as they experience uncertainty, loss and great anxiety, or as they face their own mortality or that of those they love, are too great to unravel and comprehend completely. Supporting patients like Samina and her family in Case Scenario 6.2, who all have different spiritual and religious needs, is hugely challenging, and there will always be some issues that are left unresolved. However, if practitioners are prepared to work in a person-centred and relationship-based way, are aware of their strengths and limitations, and work collaboratively within multi-disciplinary teams, spiritual care can be effectively provided. Moreover, if healthcare professionals are able to live with personal helplessness, own it and hold it (and express it to supportive others as appropriate), spiritual needs will be met as difficult questions are permitted to be voiced without answer, deep emotions are expressed and vulnerabilities are exposed in a safe, supportive and accepting context. This can make a huge difference to experience and outcome for service users, including at times a more peaceful death, and to vocational fulfilment for healthcare professionals. Helplessness as part of nurturing ourselves is explored in more depth in Chapter 11.

Reflective Activity 6.6 will allow you to explore what living with helplessness might mean in your professional practice.

Reflective Activity 6.6

Visiting Hour

In the pond of our new garden
were five orange stains, under
inches of ice. Weeks since anyone
had been there. Already by far
the most severe winter for years.
You broke the ice with a hammer.
I watched the goldfish appear,
blunt-nosed and delicately clear.

Since then so much has taken place
to distance us from what we were.
That it should come to this.
Unable to hide the horror
in my eyes, I stand helpless
by your bedside and can do no more
than wish it were simply a matter
of smashing the ice and giving you air.[3]

Having read the Stewart Conn poem above, think of times when your feelings have resonated with the partner of this patient in your healthcare role.
*   How did you deal with your feelings of helplessness?
*   To what extent did those feelings influence the way you cared for a patient and/or their loved ones in particular circumstances?

UNHEALTHY ASPECTS OF SPIRITUAL AND RELIGIOUS CARE

Consideration has been given to some of the meaningful and positive aspects of active involvement in a faith community for a person's well-being. Engagement in Reflective Activities 6.1 and 6.2 may have elicited for you the significant contributions that religious belief and belonging can make to patient experience. For example, strong belief associated with some world religions, including the understanding of an afterlife, may influence the risk of a patient with suicidal inclinations actually acting out such thoughts.[4] One depressed, terminally ill Buddhist patient, with whom one of the authors worked, did not act on his suicidal ideation as he believed that doing so would affect the form in which he would be reincarnated.

However, such reflection may also have affirmed or unearthed some aspects of religion that you consider unhelpful or unhealthy for individuals and communities. It is important to highlight some of the ways in which religious belief and involvement in some faith communities can threaten the well-being of patients, and to explore how the multi-disciplinary team can deal with these.

Crowley, a psychiatrist, and Jenkinson, a psychotherapist, have outlined some of the more extreme beliefs, which they term 'spiritual defences', that may prevent patients and carers from expressing their real self and needs:[5]

➤ submission to the 'other', or to authority, rationalised as humility *(this is different from Samina's belief in Allah's will, or the fatalistic and providential Calvinistic belief that what is for you will not pass you by)*

➤ inability or reticence with regard to forming intimate relationships with others, rationalised as the only worthwhile and necessary relationship in life being that with God

➤ lack of willingness to deal with personal or sexual needs, rationalised as ascetic practice

➤ failure to engage with the temporal and material things in life, assuming that 'God will provide.' One manifestation of this may be refusal of medicines or healthcare support, as spiritual healing or prayer may be considered sufficient.

Such expressions of belief, which clearly have a negative effect on a patient's well-being, will probably require specialist support in the form of a healthcare chaplain and/or appropriate referral to a clinical psychologist or psychiatrist. This has to be done sensitively, as patients may simply refuse to engage with such services or discharge themselves from care if they are able to do so. It may also require the multi-disciplinary team to screen visitors, with the patient's permission, thereby preventing faith community representatives from reinforcing beliefs that are counter to the patient's best interests. More commonly it is unwanted and overzealous visiting ministers and priests who are keen to support their flock who need to be denied access. This might be necessary due to patient fatigue, or due to clerical personality and dogmatic theology.

Three significant issues will be considered here in relation to certain beliefs held by elements of mainstream religions in the Western world, mainly Christianity, which can be unhealthily interpreted by patients or carers and reinforced by their faith community. Practitioners should be alert to these aspects of faith and belief which, especially at times of distress and vulnerability, need to be compassionately and competently handled. Again, referral to a specialist provider of spiritual care should be considered.

1. **The issue of sin, guilt and punishment is significant for many.** On the one hand, Christianity offers God's forgiveness for past mistakes and misdemeanours when individuals are contrite about what they have done. There is the opportunity to wipe the slate clean and begin again. This may be a comforting and hope-promoting belief. However, in some traditions guilt is hung heavily around believers' necks, and high standards of moral behaviour are expected, with the threat of eternal punishment for those who fall short of those standards. Believing that one is not worthy of forgiveness or that one's sins are so heinous that they are unforgivable is an unhealthy expression of faith.

2. **Homosexual orientation and practice.** This is considered a sin in some traditions within mainstream Christianity, while some Christians believe that homosexual orientation without being sexually active is acceptable (a 'love the sinner, hate the sin' stance). Some people who may have struggled with their sexuality for years remain in faith communities that hold such beliefs. Often they remain silent about their sexual orientation. When faced with death or illness they may reassess their lives and identity, and come to a point of crisis. Patients or carers who were brought up in or belong to such churches may find it very difficult to reconcile their sexual orientation and/or practices with their faith or the beliefs that others tell them they should have. Holding beliefs or repeatedly being reminded of beliefs which do not allow anyone to be fully who they are is not conducive to spiritual or emotional well-being.

3. **The place of anger.** Unfortunately, like many communities, cultures and families, the church does not handle anger well. Anger in many church communities is perceived as a negative emotion, and its expression is not encouraged. In fact it is actively discouraged in many quarters. As a result, some Christians will struggle to deal with any anger they feel in relation to loss, death, self, others, and especially God. Expression of anger may well be perceived as unChristian, even as a poor witness of their faith to others, when there is the expectation that adversity should be faced with so-called Christ-like courage and humility. Death and misfortune should be accepted with grace, and dying should be done peacefully and without complaint. Feelings of anger in such circumstances may be suppressed, turned inward or leak out unintentionally, affecting relationships with others, self and, ironically, with God.

CHAPLAINS OR SPECIALIST SPIRITUAL CARE PROVIDERS

Dealing with the complexity of disentangling spirituality and religion is one of the chaplain's core skills. Rather than the roots of such knowledge and skills being in an in-depth understanding of all the main world religions and humanism, the real strength is in an in-depth understanding and personal experience of how faith and beliefs, religion and spirituality can impact on our lives. It is for this reason that chaplains are required to have a 'recognised or accredited status within a mainstream faith community or belief group.'[6] From a place of personal faith and understanding we are able to journey with others and support patients, their families and staff in their spiritual and religious needs.[6]

Consider Case Scenario 6.3 below, which describes a situation that might be encountered by a chaplain or specialist spiritual care provider.

CASE SCENARIO 6.3

James is a 73-year-old man who has been admitted to a neurosurgical ward for tests following headaches, acute vomiting and blurred vision. He has been a faithful elder in his local Church of Scotland parish church for 40 years. A Highlander by birth and a shepherd by occupation, he is married to Betty, who for the last 5 years has been housebound. He is devoted to his wife as well as to his sheep, and until a few weeks ago was still actively caring for both. His father lived until he was 90, and according to James never spoke a cross word or raised his voice in earnest. He was a true Christian gentleman in James's eyes, and someone whom he always aspired to imitate.

You have been asked to see James because since being diagnosed as having an aggressive and inoperable brain tumour, he has been extremely short with and rude to the nursing staff. They are aware that this is not normal behaviour for him.

At first James is reticent about speaking to you, but after he finds out that you grew up on a farm, and that you know the difference between a Blackface and a Cheviot, he begins to open up. He is bursting with anger about how unfair his situation is. Who is going to look after Betty? What about his sheep? However, he feels immensely guilty about feeling angry, especially with God. He is mortified about his recent behaviour on the ward.

- What issues may be involved for James?
- How can you help to alleviate his spiritual distress?
- What resources from his faith tradition might you utilise to help you?

A chaplain who, while being perceived as having religious authority, gives devout believers permission to be angry with God or to question God's existence or presence, can be a powerful therapeutic tool if used appropriately. Such feelings of rage, despair and abandonment are not only biblical but Christ-like. Reading from the Psalms, Job and the Gospels may be helpful here.

Developing our awareness of what we feel about as well as what we understand by the terms 'spirituality' and 'religion' is crucial to providing person-centred care. This frees us to be open to what others believe and find meaning and purpose in, and helps us to focus on their spiritual and religious needs during their healthcare experience.

FURTHER READING

➤ Coyte ME, Gilbert P, Nicholls V. *Spirituality, Values and Mental Health: jewels for the journey*. London: Jessica Kingsley Publishers; 2007.

➤ NHS Education for Scotland. *Spiritual Care Matters: an introductory resource for all NHS Scotland staff*. Edinburgh: NHS Education for Scotland; 2009. www.nes.scot.nhs.uk/documents/publications (accessed January 2011).

➤ NHS Education for Scotland. *A Multi-Faith Resource for Healthcare Staff*. Edinburgh: NHS Education for Scotland; 2006. www.nes.scot.nhs.uk/documents/publications (accessed November 2010).

➤ Neuberger J. *Caring for Dying People of Different Faiths*, 3rd edn. Oxford: Radcliffe Publishing Ltd; 2004.

➤ Scottish Government Health Department, NHS Scotland and Scottish Inter Faith Council. *Religion and Belief Matter: an information resource for healthcare staff.* Edinburgh: Scottish Government; 2007. www.nes.scot.nhs.uk/documents/ publications (accessed November 2010).

REFERENCES

1 The Scottish Government. *Chief Executive Letter (2008) 49 – Spiritual Care.* Edinburgh: The Scottish Government Healthcare Policy and Strategy Directorate; 2008. p. 1.

2 Wright S. *Reflections on Spirituality and Health.* London: Whurr Publishers; 2005. p. 3.

3 Conn S. *Stolen Light: selected poems.* Tarset: Bloodaxe Books Ltd; 1999.

4 Salem M, Foskett J. Religion and religious experience. In: Cook C, Powell A, Sims A (eds) *Spirituality and Psychiatry.* London: Royal College of Psychiatrists Publications; 2009. pp. 233–53.

5 Crowley N, Jenkinson G. Pathological spirituality. In: Cook C, Powell A, Sims A (eds) *Spirituality and Psychiatry.* London: Royal College of Psychiatrists Publications; 2009. p. 255.

6 UK Board of Healthcare Chaplaincy. *Spiritual and Religious Care Capabilities and Competences for Healthcare Chaplains. 4.2.3.* Cambridge: UK Board of Healthcare Chaplaincy; 2009.

CHAPTER 7

Spiritual assessment

INTRODUCTION

In previous chapters we have been exploring spirituality through a process of self-awareness and developing and understanding of the elements that contribute to a person's spirituality, such as faith, belief and culture, and recognising spiritual distress. Once we understand the breadth and depth of what spirituality can be, we are then in a place to consider assessment. How do you assess a person's spiritual needs?

There is a small body of opinion that spirituality is an aspect of the patient's private life, and that spiritual assessment and care should be left to chaplains (i.e. those with expertise in spiritual and religious care).[1] However, in contrast, there is an overwhelming body of opinion – in professional standards, guidelines and competences, in World Health Organization statements, and in NHS standards and guidelines – that firmly roots spiritual care within the healthcare practice of all healthcare professionals:

> The provision of spiritual care by NHS staff is not yet another demand on their hard-pressed time. It is the very essence of their work, and it enables and promotes healing in the fullest sense to all parties, both giver and receiver.[2]

This general consensus asserts that 'spiritual care matters' and is integral to healthcare. How and when it should be assessed, and by whom, engenders a wide-ranging debate. This chapter will refer to this debate and offer some basic guidance for readers to use in their various clinical settings and professional practice.

STRUCTURING SPIRITUAL ASSESSMENT

Linked to the argument for a standardised working definition of spirituality are proposals for a generic spiritual assessment tool that can be incorporated into healthcare practice. McSherry and Ross, long-time advocates of such a view, draw together contributions from experienced practitioners to debate spiritual assessment in depth, and conclude that no one tool holds the answer.[3] Instead they suggest that the key to spiritual assessment lies in the personal and professional gifts and skills of healthcare practitioners, a mix of formal and informal assessment, and recognising that it is as much an art as a science. The authors draw the same conclusions. The chapters in this book have been developed to support this broad view of spiritual assessment and care, and to encourage healthcare professionals to increase their knowledge and skills so that they can become the person-centred 'quality carers' that McSherry and Ross envisage.

Reflective Activity 7.1 will encourage you to reflect on your experiences of spiritual assessment in your current professional practice.

Reflective Activity 7.1

Reflect on your experiences of spiritual assessment by answering the following questions:
- In what ways do you currently assess patients' spiritual needs?
  - Are there specific questions in the admissions process?
  - Is there a structured spiritual assessment tool?
  - What personal skills would you use to assess and discern spiritual need?
- How would a patient's spiritual needs be assessed and communicated within the healthcare team?
  - Does one professional group (i.e. nurses) make the assessment or do all contribute?
  - Are spiritual needs discussed at team meetings?
  - Are spiritual needs and actions taken recorded in the patient records?

Hopefully our current experiences of spiritual assessment will go beyond the old traditional 'one-question' model of spiritual assessment, namely 'What religion are you?' Developments in care, including the introduction of care pathways such as the Liverpool Care Pathway, often include spiritual assessment and make a difference to patient care.[4] In specialist areas where issues of significant loss and death are a daily facet of care, such as transplant units, neonatal care and palliative care, spiritual assessment will be more routine and in-depth, and should have dedicated specialist support from chaplaincy services.

ASSESSMENT TOOLS

Spiritual care does not lend itself to a traditional questionnaire-style assessment tool where there are simple 'yes/no' answers. By nature assessment tools are developed to be simple and quick to use. However, there is a risk that the patient's spirituality will then conform to the tool, rather than the healthcare professional being enabled to conduct a meaningful spiritual assessment that can in turn open up a meaningful conversation. In contrast, a number of tools have been developed that make use of narrative and encouraging the patient to 'tell their story'. These tools require healthcare professionals to develop good communication skills and draw on their instinct and experience. However, these tools sometimes make assumptions about the relationship between spirituality and religion that can sidetrack our assessment along religious routes if used rigidly.

The FICA tool developed by Post, Puchalski and Larson is one such example.[5] It focuses on four aspects of assessment, each containing questions that can be used and adapted to our own style and cultural setting:

➤ Faith: *'What do you believe in that gives meaning to your life?'*
➤ Importance and influence: *'How important is your faith (or religion or spirituality) to you?'*
➤ Community: *'Are you a part of a religious or spiritual community?'*
➤ Address or Application: *'How would you like me to address these issues in your health care?' 'How can we assist you in your spiritual care?'*

A similar format is used by Anandarajah and Hight in the HOPE tool,[6] where the user can create questions around each of the four areas of this acronym:

➤ H – sources of Hope, strength, comfort, meaning, peace, love and connection
➤ O – the role of Organised religion in the life of the patient
➤ P – Personal spirituality and practices
➤ E – the Effects on medical care and end-of-life decisions.

The difficulty that the authors have with these tools is the way in which religion features early on in the assessment. In the authors' experience, if you ask religious questions at the beginning of a spiritual assessment, you will get 'religious' answers to all of the spiritual questions. One tool that uses the same conversational style of assessment yet allows for a patient-focused spiritual response has been offered by Jackson.[7] Although originally developed for palliative care, the questions in this tool can be adapted and reworded for use in any healthcare setting:

> *'When you were admitted you gave us a lot of information. We asked you about how you were feeling. How are you feeling now?'*

> Depending on the answer, the following questions might be asked:

> ➤ *'How easy is it for you to find hope and peace in your life at the moment?'*
> ➤ *'What makes it difficult for you at the moment?'*
> ➤ *'What changes has your illness brought about?'*
> ➤ *'Do you pray or meditate? Does it help you find meaning in life or not?'*

Such assessment tools that engage the patient in conversation can lead us into the realms of spiritual assessment. However, their strength lies in their adaptability rather than in offering a clear and usable generic tool.

WHEN SHOULD SPIRITUAL ASSESSMENT TAKE PLACE?

If we accept that spiritual care is an integral part of all healthcare practice as outlined in the NHS Education for Scotland resource *Spiritual Care Matters*, there is an argument for including spiritual assessment in the general admissions procedures.[8] Such a move could ensure that spiritual care is not overlooked or avoided, and would lend itself to audit. However, it could also serve to reduce spiritual care to the kind of tick-box assessment that we criticised earlier.

Case Scenario 7.1 and Reflective Activity 7.2 will demonstrate the difficulties of deciding when is the best time for a spiritual assessment to take place.

CASE SCENARIO 7.1

Mark is being admitted to the ward for investigations. He is suffering from persistent nausea and diarrhoea. After his details have been taken and his physical symptoms have been assessed, Mark is asked if he is aware of any spiritual needs that he has at this time and replies 'No, I can't get my head round any of that, I've been like this for days and the toilet is all I can think of.' Three days later Mark's nausea and diarrhoea appear to be under control with medication, but the cause is still unclear and is being investigated. Although Mark responds well to the staff and appears bright and good-humoured, when on his own he seems withdrawn and has a sad expression on his face. While monitoring Mark's vital signs his nurse, Evelyn, says to him: 'Mark, I notice when you're on your own you seem sad. I get the sense you've got something on your mind. Can you tell me what you've been thinking about?' Mark is quiet for a moment and says nothing. Evelyn completes her tasks and follows up with a tentative question: 'I have a few minutes just now to talk. Can you tell me what's on your mind?' Mark discloses that he recently heard that he may lose his job. His wife suffers from depression and he's really worried that this news will 'set her off' again. On top of that he says he has two children at university, who get no grant or help with their fees and accommodation, and are therefore dependent on him. It's giving him a constant knot in his stomach and he can't think about anything else.

Reflective Activity 7.2

Reflecting on Case Scenario 7.1 and drawing on your own clinical experience, answer the following questions:
- Would a more in-depth spiritual assessment on admission have been helpful to Mark?
  - If not, or if you are unsure, when in your clinical setting would be the best time to assess?
- Would a structured spiritual assessment a few days after admission such as that suggested by Jackson[7] be useful in this case?
  - What would you ask as an opening question to begin such an assessment?

There is no one correct answer in this scenario, nor is there one best time to conduct a spiritual assessment. There is a good chance that Mark's spiritual distress is contributing to or may indeed be the cause of his physical symptoms, in which case a more in-depth assessment that went beyond his physical symptoms could have helped. It is also just as likely that the nature of Mark's physical symptoms was so all-consuming that he couldn't 'get his head round any of that' when asked about his spiritual needs on admission.

There is no 'ideal' time at which to assess. There are arguments for assessing on admission, after three days, or even every few days, as patients can change from day to day or from hour to hour. While structured assessments at particular times are good screening tools, the authors take the view that continuous spiritual assessment is the only reliable form of assessment. If healthcare professionals have the knowledge and skills to recognise the signs of spiritual distress, this can be integrated into everyday practice and therefore facilitate continuous assessment. This view was developed in Chapter 5 when appraising competence in spiritual care.

INSTINCT AND EXPERIENCE

Although spiritual assessment tools can be useful, an in-depth and meaningful spiritual assessment rests more on a combination of our personal discernment and experience combined with good communication skills, as outlined in Chapter 3. In Case Scenario 7.1 above, it is Evelyn's instinct and experience that allow her to pick up on Mark's spiritual distress – a mixture of what she saw in his facial expression, the way he appeared different when on his own, and knowing that anxiety and worry can present with similar physical symptoms. There might have been a number of other factors we don't know about that sparked Evelyn's gut feeling to respond. For example:

➤ Mark's reaction to the medication might have been different from the norm
➤ he may have appeared particularly withdrawn after visiting time
➤ he may not have been eating anything, not even the food that patients might want to try even with nausea.

As a rule of thumb, if an internal niggle – something in our gut – seems to be saying that something is amiss, the likelihood is that we are right. The danger at such times is that we assume what the patient might be thinking or feeling, and this is where there is value in spiritual assessment and a spiritual assessment tool that uses open questions and helps to prompt the patient to respond.

Reflective Activity 7.3 will guide you to reflect on your instinct and experience and how you might develop your skills in spiritual assessment.

Reflective Activity 7.3

From your own clinical experience, recall a case where as a result of your discernment and experience you sensed that there was likely to be some underlying psychological, social or spiritual need in a patient for whom you were caring. Reflect on the following questions:
- Describe what you saw or heard that made you think or sense that there was such a need. For example:

(continued)

- something that the patient said or didn't say
- something in the patient's demeanour
- something in the patient's reaction to others.
- How did your instinct present itself to you? For example:
  - a gut feeling inside
  - a niggling thought in your mind
  - something that wouldn't go away.
- How would you normally respond to your instinct? For example:
  - act on it immediately
  - mull it over
  - check it with a colleague.
- Would you respond differently at different times? How would you respond in the following scenarios?
  - You are busy with other patients and don't have time just now.
  - You have only a few minutes just now, but would have more time later.
  - Having 'asked the question' you quickly realise that you have opened up a significant issue that will take considerable skill and time to deal with.

Self-awareness of how we can recognise and respond to our instinct and experience is a valuable tool in spiritual assessment. It is remarkable what can be achieved in the way of spiritual assessment in just a few minutes with a skilful opening question asked at the right time. However, we also need to have a strategy for dealing with whatever arises once we have opened the door. Time is an ever-present pressure, and there can be a sense of fear of the unknown. Will something familiar be raised which we have experience of or will it be something that takes us by surprise and is way beyond our expertise? The key is to have a strategy for dealing with the restrictions on our time, and when something unexpected or complex arises. It is always acceptable to say to a patient 'That sounds like something significant we should talk about. Can I come back later when I have some more time?' or 'I appreciate that was difficult to say. I have a colleague who has more experience in this area. Is it OK if I ask them to come and speak with you?'

Spiritual care does not lend itself to a structured process undertaken in only one encounter or rely on a single tool to be effective. Although assessment tools can be useful in suggesting ways in which healthcare professionals can engage patients and their family carers in meaningful conversations, they are not an end in themselves. There is no ideal time at which to assess spiritual needs. It will vary from one setting to another and from one patient to another. A process of continuous assessment can be achieved by healthcare professionals who have a knowledge and understanding of spiritual needs and how they are manifested, and who use their discernment and experience to guide them. These issues are discussed in more detail in Chapter 5.

CHAPLAIN OR SPIRITUAL CARE PROFESSIONAL

There are a number of factors that influence our understanding of and views on spiritual assessment. By its very nature, spiritual assessment needs to be a flexible process to enable it to respond to the changing needs of patients and their family/carers. Also, as chaplaincy moves from a model of ward rounds, where every patient received a visit, to one that relies more on referral, spiritual assessment becomes more important, as it is the means by which informed and appropriate referrals will be made.

Although there is a considerable literature on spiritual assessment in healthcare journals and textbooks, little has been written by chaplains themselves. In contrast, however, there is considerable anecdotal evidence to suggest that chaplains are being creative in encouraging spiritual assessment and are working across traditional professional boundaries. For example, in one mental health setting it is the occupational therapists who conduct the spiritual assessments. The chaplain recognised that the questions which the occupational therapists were asking in their assessment were on the same themes as a spiritual assessment – for example, the impact that the patient's illness was having on their life at home, and how they were coping. A training session on identifying and assessing spiritual needs was arranged with the occupational therapists, who grasped the similarities in their approach and how it could be adapted to meet both assessments. As a result, the chaplaincy department is receiving an increased number of informed referrals and is able to direct its resources appropriately.

Given the diverse range of services that can exist within an acute hospital, it is likely that no one form of assessment will suit all, and a variety of forms of assessment might be in place. Reflective Activities 7.4 and 7.5 will help you to consider the ways in which spiritual care is assessed in your clinical setting, and their effectiveness.

Reflective Activity 7.4

Drawing on your own clinical experience, critically appraise your local arrangements for spiritual assessment and the protocols for referral to the chaplaincy service. You may find it helpful to consider the following:

- What staff group or profession conducts initial spiritual assessments?
- When is the spiritual assessment conducted? Does it take place on admission or at another time?
- Are referrals mainly informal (in the passing) or do they use the protocol for referral to the chaplaincy service?
- How often are the referrals 'informed' and specific rather than non-specific? For example, *'Jean has been very quiet for the last couple of days, and gets upset when her family have visited. I think that she's needing to talk more, and I said I'd ask you to visit'* rather than *'Jean isn't great today – could you have a word?'*

Given the diversity that exists in larger hospitals, you may find it helpful to revisit this activity for different departments and specialties within your hospital. Even within a small unit you may find that there are differences between wards that could highlight good practice and be adapted as a model for service improvement. Audit is a useful tool and can provide evidence for good practice. Reflective Activity 7.5 gives an example of how service standards can be used as a basis for audit to support spiritual assessment and referral protocols, and to identify training needs.

Reflective Activity 7.5

Consider conducting an audit of spiritual assessment and the referrals made to the chaplaincy service. You may find that you have access to a hospital clinical audit facilitator who will be able to help and advise you. You might consider an audit of the following:

- Spiritual assessment from *Standard 1 Spiritual and Religious Care.*[9]
- Referral protocols from *Standard 2 Access to Chaplaincy Services.*[2]
- Referrals to the chaplaincy service:
  - Which wards refer more than others?
  - Are there any wards that rarely refer?
  - Are the referrals informed (with reasons) or generic, in response to an admissions question such as 'Do you want to see the chaplain?'?

Such an audit could highlight strengths and weaknesses in spiritual assessment, identify areas of good practice, and be used to develop training and support for areas where there is a need for improvement and change. Implementing change is rarely easy. However, if the rationale for change is supported by audit and evidence from practice it is much easier to initiate.

Spiritual assessment is by nature a flexible and fluid process that requires knowledge, skill, instinct and experience. Although assessment tools can be valuable, how and when they are used and most effective is open to debate. It is unlikely that any one tool will be of universal value. However, a flexible tool that uses open questions which can be adapted to local or departmental needs and culture can be effective. These different components of spiritual assessment are explored in more detail elsewhere in this book when considering communication, competence, disentangling spiritual and religious care, and responding to spiritual and religious needs.

FURTHER READING

➤ Gordon T, Mitchell D. Making sense of spiritual care. In: Kinghorn S, Gaines S (eds) *Palliative Nursing*, 2nd edn. Edinburgh: Bailliere Tindall; 2007.

REFERENCES

1 Randall F, Downie RS. *Palliative Care Ethics: a good companion*. Oxford: Oxford University Press; 1996.

2 UK Board of Healthcare Chaplaincy. *Standards for NHS Chaplaincy Services*. Cambridge: UK Board of Healthcare Chaplaincy; 2009. p. 4.

3 McSherry W, Ross L (eds). *Spiritual Assessment in Healthcare Practice*. Keswick: M&K Publishing; 2010.

4 Ellershaw J, Wilkinson S. *Care of the Dying: a pathway to excellence*. Oxford: Oxford University Press; 2010.

5 Post SG, Puchalski C, Larson D. Physicians and patient spirituality: professional boundaries, competency, and ethics. *Annals of Internal Medicine* 2000; **133:** 748–9.

6 Anandarajah G, Hight E. Spirituality and medical practice: using the HOPE questions as a practical tool for spiritual assessment. *American Family Physician* 2001; **63:** 81–8.

7 Jackson J. The challenge of providing spiritual care. *Professional Nurse* 2004; **20:** 24–6.

8 NHS Education for Scotland. *Spiritual Care Matters: an introductory resource for all NHS Scotland staff*. Edinburgh: NHS Education for Scotland; 2009.

9 UK Board of Healthcare Chaplaincy. *Standards for NHS Chaplaincy Services*, op. cit., p. 3.

CHAPTER 8

Responding to spiritual and religious needs

INTRODUCTION

The majority of healthcare provision is task-oriented. This is often a matter of pragmatic necessity. A doctor needs to take a patient's history, perform a physical examination, make differential diagnoses and organise relevant investigations in order to make a definitive diagnosis. Nurses are required to perform an array of tasks when looking after the physical and mental well-being of the patients in their care. Allied healthcare professionals and social workers have to carry out a range of assessments in order to decide what physical, social and financial support might best help those with whom they work. In contrast, the spiritual component of healthcare is counter-cultural, as it is predominantly person-centred. Sometimes, in our busy and complex healthcare systems, process and procedure can take precedence over the needs of patient, carers and indeed staff. Encouragingly, however, under recent government guidance many healthcare services are seeking to enable their staff to provide more person-centred care. For example, the Scottish Government has recently developed a quality strategy which requires Scottish health boards to re-orient their services in this way.[1]

Meeting service users' actual spiritual and religious needs rather than their assumed needs means paying due respect and attention to their particular story, told their way. Fundamental to all person-centred healthcare, including spiritual and religious care, is respect for another's dignity, life-position, beliefs and values – in other words, their uniqueness as a human being. In addition, respect for another's understanding of their experience, wherever they are on their journey through life, and no matter how much their frame of reference resonates with or differs from that of the practitioner, is crucial. In the context of palliative care, Irish chaplain John Quinlan has expressed it as follows:[2]

> Our task is to stay with people in their fear and free them. They are living persons – living towards death as you and I are, even if we are at a different stage of the journey. Always treat them as the living persons they are.

The following activity will help you to reflect on different aspects of what it means to be human in relationship with others. It is particularly relevant as we consider relating to patients, their loved ones and colleagues in contemporary healthcare settings where technology and efficiency are so highly valued. In such potentially dehumanising environments, respecting the uniqueness of others can become a lower priority.

Reflective Activity 8.1

Read Kathy Galloway's poem *Real* slowly out loud. Allow yourself time to dwell on any aspects that resonate or jar for you.[3]

I'm not a symbol
I'm not a statistic
I'm not the inches in somebody's column.

I'm not admirable, but
I'm not pitiable either.
I'm simply human.

If you turned me inside out,
You'd find fury, fear, regret and sorrow
Struggling with the love and the longing,
Hope and wonder,
And all my neediness.

Please take these things seriously.
Don't pietize or glamorize or trivalize or sermonize.
They are marks of my life,
Gift and loss,
Wound and offence.
Please respect them.

I am at odds with all that requires me to be a symbol.
I insist on being real.

- How does this poem make you feel about the way others relate to you and your individual life story at work and in your personal life?
- How real do we allow patients to be in our healthcare system? Think especially of your place of work.
- To what extent are patients respected for what they are rather than what our healthcare system wants them to be or to conform to?
- How do you relate to patients and carers?

COPING WITH ILL HEALTH, INJURY, ACCIDENT OR DEATH

It seems obvious that human beings all deal with life's major challenges and tragedies in different ways. There are no right or wrong ways. Person-centred spiritual care has to be open to how patients and their carers are dealing with what is happening in their lives in a manner that is appropriate for them. One of the great dangers in healthcare is paternalism – that is, practitioners assuming they know what is best for an individual or family and trying to fix things for them. Spiritual care is not about patching up broken lives or sticking a plaster over a wound. On the contrary, it is often about holding tensions and paradoxes while supporting service users as they struggle to find meaning or the resources within themselves or around them to deal with their situation. At its best, spiritual care involves empowering others to live with, and through, anxiety and distress in a manner that feels right for them. In the provision of spiritual care, healthcare staff need to remember that the suffering or pain endured by another is not the practitioner's to decide how to deal with. Options or opportunities for support should only be offered, never imposed. 'Doing to' or 'deciding for' is not best practice. Accepting the way that others cope with situations can be difficult, especially if we feel that we would act in another way or that the coping mechanism that has been chosen is less than helpful.

The following activity will enable you to reflect on the coping mechanisms of others, how they differ from one individual to another, and how as a person and as a healthcare professional you react to how others deal with stress and anxiety.

Reflective Activity 8.2

The Scottish poet Hugh MacDiarmid writes of a scenario with which those working in paediatrics will be very familiar.[4] However, his poem *The Two Parents* is worth reading by all seeking to support others who are dealing with illness, loss or anticipated death.

I love my little son, and yet when he was ill
I could not confine myself to his bedside.
I was impatient of his squalid little needs,
His laboured breathing and the fretful way he cried
And longed for my wide range of interests again,
Whereas his mother sank without another care
To that dread level of nothing but life itself
And stayed day and night, till he was better, there.

Women may pretend, yet they always dismiss
Everything but mere being just like this.

- Which of the two parents do you relate to most? Why?
- Do either of their actions trouble you? Why?
- What issues may be involved for them as a family and individually?
- How would you approach offering support to them?
- What kind of issues might you have to address with them as a couple, or individually, for their collective and personal well-being?

In the above poem, two parents who both love their child are dealing with his illness in different ways. A father who is struggling with his own helplessness and the fragility of his son desires activity and involvement in the normality of his usual daily routine. Moreover, he is perhaps not only fearful for his son's mortality, but also starkly reminded of his own. His wife, in contrast, focuses all of her attention on being with her son. She offers him her constant presence and energy, investing everything she has in being with him. These two parents are part of the same family, yet their spiritual needs will be different.

A family may describe itself as, for example, Sikh or Anglican, but each individual will practise their faith, if at all, in a variety of ways because they are influenced by cultural or societal norms differently. Gender differences, as shown in Reflective Activity 8.2, may significantly influence how people cope with adversity, as does belonging to different generations.

RESOURCES AVAILABLE TO PRACTITIONERS IN THE PROVISION OF SPIRITUAL CARE

There are three main resources available to help us as healthcare practitioners to provide person-centred spiritual care:
➤ relevant up-to-date information
➤ the expertise, experience and abilities of others
➤ ourselves.

The rest of this chapter will focus on exploring these resources. The reader should bear in mind that underpinning the sensitive utilisation of these tools is the desire to empower service users to deal with their situation in the manner that they find most helpful.

SPIRITUAL CARE AS ENABLING CHOICE

One of the most difficult issues that patients and their carers face when dealing with illness, injury, accident and hospitalisation is a lack of control over important elements of their lives. This is a huge loss. Moreover, it has to be coped with at the same time as they are dealing with other possible losses, such loss of dignity, role, identity, orientation and structure to life, body image and function (spiritual care and loss will be explored more fully in Chapter 10). A significant aspect of person-centred spiritual and religious care involves enabling the patient to regain some form of control by offering them choice as to how their needs may be met. Such choice, depending on service user needs, might include whether:
➤ they wish our company at that particular moment (or at another time, if possible), whether to talk or not or if they want the company of a colleague who is better equipped to deal with their particular spiritual needs
➤ they wish to see a representative from their faith or belief group or not (this may take the form of a request for particular prayers or rituals)

➤ they would like access to the quiet room/sanctuary/prayer room
➤ they require any resources to help them to practise their faith or beliefs (e.g. sacred texts, prayer beads or a mat) or to help them to relax (e.g. relaxation tapes or appropriate music)
➤ they would like to attend any services of worship that may take place in the hospital or hospice.

It is crucial to remember, therefore, that patients and their carers choose who (if anyone) they wish to confide in and seek spiritual and emotional support from. It is important that this is not only respected but positively encouraged. Often service users observe how members of staff relate not just to themselves but to other patients, relatives and each other in a clinical context. Spiritual care is best provided within a relationship of trust, and individuals will select someone whom they feel they can confide in and with whom they can share their concerns, 'why' questions and inner wrestling. Commonly patients trust their souls to those to whom they trust their bodies. Patients often open up to those who wash them and toilet them, who tend their wounds and help them develop their physical strength and mobility. Patients also often share their spiritual and emotional selves when performing other tasks, such as dressing or stair practice.

Healthcare professionals should also never underestimate the spiritual care that is provided by members of a patient's family, their friends, other patients and visitors. Single rooms may reduce the rate of hospital-acquired infections, but they also reduce the emotional and spiritual support that patients and their carers may provide for one another. Spiritual care is as much shared in community settings as it is offered in one-to-one relationships. Loneliness and isolation play a large part in contributing to spiritual dis-ease or distress. Making meaningful connections with fellow patients or carers, whether about football, families or exploring existential angst, can help to alleviate this as well as build morale and self-worth. Where possible, choice should be offered to patients, whether they would prefer a single or shared room or ward, or given gentle encouragement, where appropriate, to move bed spaces if company and conversation, or indeed solitude and space, are perceived to be of potential benefit.

INFORMATION SHARING

To enable patients to make informed choices, practitioners need to be up to date with the appropriate information about support or advice available, and discerning about when is the right time to share it, and how to do so. Sharing information about sources of spiritual and religious support, or offering bench-marking examples to explain the options that are open to patients and carers, is important. However, this has to be done when those involved have the time, energy and resources to explain as well as to listen to, and absorb, at least some of what is said. In addition to sharing information and normalising examples of feelings and behaviours orally (e.g. following bereavement), best practice is also to give patients and their carers the same information in written form. This enables them to revisit what was initially said, or indeed to read through it several times, and it helps to facilitate the process of understanding and digesting information. As a result, the likelihood of informed decisions being made during times of loss and distress is increased.

The following case scenario will help you to reflect on these issues. It is set in the context of a baby's death on a maternity unit. It is an example of how timely and sensitive information sharing can enable service users to make informed choices and can thus help to meet their spiritual needs in times of confusion and uncertainty.

CASE SCENARIO 8.1

Sadly, Joe and Heidi's first baby has been stillborn at 37 weeks of gestation. Heidi had not felt the baby move for a day or two and, unfortunately, at her doctor's surgery the heartbeat could not be traced either. Heidi was referred to the local maternity unit where it was confirmed that her baby was dead. She was admitted the following day, at her request, to induce her labour. Prior to labour being induced the midwife who was looking after the family asked if Joe and Heidi would like some information about what would happen after delivery and the choices that they might like to make about marking their baby's life and death, as well as certain practical arrangements they would have to consider. Fear of the unknown was a big part of their distress at that time, so even though the whole scenario seemed so unreal, they agreed.

Hazel, their midwife, then talked to them about labour and the option of seeing and holding their baby after delivery. Joe and Heidi agreed to see Matthew, the chaplain (once Hazel had reassured them he was not there to 'give them religion' but to help them make the decisions that were right for them and their baby), when Heidi was in the early part of labour. Matthew sensitively introduced information about the practical arrangements that Joe and Heidi were legally obliged to make and how they might mark the uniqueness and special nature of their baby according to their beliefs, experience and worldview. Leaflets relating to these issues and regarding choices about involvement in funeral arrangements were left with the couple.

Jody was delivered 26 hours later. Following her birth, Joe and Heidi spent a short time with Jody but Heidi was too exhausted both physically and emotionally to talk much with anyone. After having a sleep, a shower and something to eat, Joe and Heidi asked to see Matthew again. Not only did he answer their questions about the options for Jody's disposal and registering her stillbirth but also he shared examples of what other parents had chosen to do, or not do, in similar circumstances. He was also able to refer to recent research carried out on baby death and parental experience. All of this information helped to normalise the couple's feelings and experience while at the same time giving them an idea of social norms as a benchmark for their decision making. Neither Joe nor Heidi had any previous experience of the death of someone close to them, let alone the death of a baby. Before Matthew left he gave them not only information about bereavement support, including

(continued)

websites that other parents had found helpful but also his contact telephone number and the hours he was available should they wish to get in touch with him.

Three days later, after registering Jody's stillbirth and visiting an undertaker of their choice, Joe and Heidi telephoned Matthew to ask if he would help them to plan and conduct a short funeral service for Jody, during which they wanted her to be cremated.

Reflective Activity 8.3 allows you to think about how you share information to enable patients and their carers to make informed choices as part of the spiritual and religious care that you provide.

Reflective Activity 8.3

Think about the information that you give to patients and their carers to enable them to make informed choices about how they deal with an aspect of their health which includes their spiritual well-being. Reflect on:

- the timing of the sharing of information
- who shares the information
- how they share it
- where they share it
- any training or support that is given regarding this area of care.

For example, after a death, what are the procedures in your workplace with regard to sharing information about what practical actions the relatives will have to take and how they do so?

- How are relatives made aware of the normal feelings that they may experience in the days and weeks ahead and what support may be available to them should they become concerned about themselves or someone else in the family?
- Are relatives given information about making funeral arrangements and the details of those who might help them with this?

If patients or their carers are receiving information which will be significant to them when they are at home, it is also important that they feel they have permission to get in touch again if they need something clarified or explained further. Therefore a contact telephone number and the name of a contact person, where possible, should be given.

Referral to competent and capable others

Healthcare staff are the gatekeepers to specialist spiritual care provision. Therefore, as outlined in Chapter 5, it is important that practitioners are aware of the role of chaplains (which includes supporting healthcare colleagues while they provide spiritual care to patients and carers in difficult situations), when referral to them is appropriate, and how to make such a referral.

Members of local faith and belief groups can be a tremendously valuable resource in terms of providing spiritual as well as religious care. However, healthcare practitioners should never assume that just because a patient or carer states an affiliation with a faith community or belief group, they necessarily want a visit from a representative (*see also* Chapters 6 and 7). They should always be given a choice. Nor, indeed, should we assume that because a person's religious needs have been responded to, all of their spiritual needs will also have been met (as was explored in Case Scenario 6.1). Many faith communities provide visitors or befrienders who support vulnerable and lonely people in their own homes, in healthcare institutions and in care homes. They can provide continuity of support before and during admission as well as after discharge. Such visitors and their faith leaders may help healthcare professionals to contextualise a patient's condition and give a realistic appraisal of their home life and local support mechanisms. At times they can also act as a patient's advocate when the family is scattered or absent.

Both sharing information and referring service users to specialist spiritual care providers are tasks which are an important part of the spiritual and religious care that is offered within the health service. However, more challenging is spiritual care, which primarily involves 'being with', listening to and accompanying the patient, their carers and colleagues, rather than 'talking to' or 'doing things for' them. Here the personhood and natural abilities of the practitioner are of greatest importance in embodying and performing the art of spiritual care.

SELF AS THE MOST SIGNIFICANT RESOURCE

Whatever the level of competency at which a healthcare worker is providing spiritual and religious care (as described in detail in Chapter 5), the authors believe that the most important tool which practitioners have at their disposal is themselves. At the core of such provision it is not so much what is said or done that is significant but how it is said and the manner in which a task is performed. Spiritual care is about the quality of the relationship formed with patients and their carers by a practitioner, which is essentially the healthcare professional's way of being with them and relating to them. Thus spiritual care is not just an activity that is added on to the physical, social and psychological dimensions of healthcare, but rather it is how these aspects of care are carried out. It is our humanity and willingness to share ourselves as we are – not just our clinical acumen, technical excellence or diagnostic ability – that enhances patient experience and outcome. In fact, in many situations our self is the most effective, if not only, therapeutic tool that we have. Being human and open with another gives them permission, especially if they feel vulnerable and anxious (as most patients and carers naturally do), to be as they really are and express themselves as they need to.

It is within such developing relationships of trust that a service user's spiritual and religious needs can be most appropriately assessed.

Each healthcare professional makes the choice as to how much of self is shared or revealed in any encounter, task performed or indeed in the vocational role embodied. This of course may vary from one day to another, and even from one situation to another, depending on the practitioner's sense of well-being and the particular circumstances and the other(s) involved. As healthcare practitioners we are as human as the people we seek to care for, so there are times when we need to distance ourselves from certain situations, patients and families in order to look after ourselves. However, for many healthcare professionals the *normal* pattern whereby they engage with others is at a distance – keeping patients, families and colleagues at arm's length. This is commonly done by hiding their humanity and anxiety behind procedures, tasks, techniques and ritual, especially if they are threatened by exposure to uncertainty, paradox, loss or strong emotion. Such patterns of behaviour not only prevent staff having to deal with the messiness and tensions in others' lives, but also keep at bay, consciously or more likely unconsciously, the risk of being reminded of the vulnerability and fragmentation in our own lives.

Not only is it very challenging to provide person-centred spiritual care from a distance, but also it is difficult to adequately assess spiritual and religious need in order to make a referral to another whose natural ability is to provide the compassion, empathy and discernment required. On the other hand, if we become totally immersed in the pain and anguish of others, we risk rendering ourselves overwhelmed and incapacitated, with the danger of burnout if such behaviour is normative. It is the fine line that we tread at times between distancing ourselves from, and drowning in, the suffering of others which necessitates reflection on practice, supervision or mentoring and personal discernment to maintain healthy helpful therapeutic relationships and balance for ourselves.

Case Scenario 8.2 will allow you to begin to explore ways of being and relating.

CASE SCENARIO 8.2

John is a 62-year-old single man who has been in a side room on a surgical ward for three weeks. He is a longstanding diabetic, a lifelong smoker and a heavy drinker. He has had an above-knee amputation on his right leg in the past. Vascular surgery on his left leg has failed, and now the toes on his left foot are turning gangrenous. John also has hospital-acquired MRSA. He has no close family and few visitors. He has recently become tearful and is very aware of further impending losses and his isolation. His behaviour and attitude towards staff can be erratic, and as a result he has been labelled on the ward as a 'difficult' patient.

Reflective Activity 8.4

Imagine that in your healthcare role you have regular contact with John to perform a routine task with him.

- How do you relate to people like John in your daily work? (Go back to your response to a similar question in Reflective Activity 8.1.)
- How does your multi-disciplinary team relate to such patients?
- How do service users respond to the way that you relate to them as you go about your daily work?
- Why do you feel this is so?

Perhaps you might like to ask a trusted individual at work about their observations of the way you relate to different types of patients or carers.

SELF-AWARENESS REVISITED

In Chapter 1 the significance of self-awareness in delivering spiritual care was highlighted. It is important here to return to the issue of reflexivity. For any practitioner, when offering spiritual care or indeed when deciding not to, it is crucial to consider whose need is being met – the practitioner's or that of the service user. And, in any situation, it is important for the practitioner to consider whether he or she is the best person to deliver what is required.

In many instances a patient or carer may already have selected you as the person they want with them at that point in time, or they may consider you to be the most appropriate person in the multi-disciplinary team to talk to. However, there are times when healthcare professionals attempt to offer care that they are not equipped to deliver (through lack of self-awareness), or seek to offer care because of their own need. Often such encounters end up focusing more on the practitioner's needs than on those of the service user (one more extreme example of this is found in Case Scenario 2.2). This is far from best or ethical practice. It is important that practitioners are aware of the position of power and responsibility that they are in when seeking to meet the spiritual needs of vulnerable people, who often will not question decisions that staff make. There is what has been described as a 'shadow side to caring',[5] of which all practitioners should be aware.

Case Scenario 8.3 is an example of a practitioner whose motivation for delivering spiritual care in the way that she did called into question whose needs were being met by the service she provided.

CASE SCENARIO 8.3

Edith was relatively new in healthcare chaplaincy. In the early hours of the morning she was called into the acute hospital where she worked to be with Joan and Ben, whose husband and father, Harry, was dying. Edith spent some time with the family while they sat at the bedside of Harry, who was unconscious. She helped Joan and Ben to share stories about him and to talk about their happy memories of their loved one, as well as their regrets and feelings about Harry's impending death. It was a time of openness and some potential healing as old hurts were discussed and previous assumptions were dealt with. However, the minutes passed into hours as Edith stayed with the family while they waited. When the breakfast trolley came round several hours later, Edith was still there. It took a polite but firm ward sister to tease Edith away by stating that the family might like some time on their own, and surely Edith now needed some rest and something to eat.

Later that day Edith popped in and out of the ward several times to see the family, and although they were polite, Edith sensed that they were rather more distant than they had been earlier. Harry died that evening.

Reflective Activity 8.5

- What might have influenced Edith's motivation to remain with this family for such a long period?
- How might Edith have supported this family differently – in a more appropriate way for them, for herself, and perhaps for the rest of the healthcare team?

CASE SCENARIO 8.3 CONTINUED

A few days later, Mary, the lead chaplain, invited Edith into her office for a coffee. After asking Edith how she was doing, Mary told her that the sister of the ward where Edith had spent so much time recently had spoken to her discretely about Edith's behaviour. The family whom Edith had supported had commented when they left that her care had been appreciated but they expressed concern about her ongoing well-being if she continued to work with others in the way she had supported them.

With some gentle encouragement, Edith talked about her need to perform well and to make her mark in the chaplaincy team as well as in the wider healthcare team. She also described how when her father was dying at home the local minister had been noticeable by his absence – apart from a quick prayer and an equally rapid exit. This had made a deep impression on her.

Reflective Activity 8.6

For all healthcare practitioners
- Think of times when, in retrospect, you have realised that your motivation for how you offered care or failed to deliver optimal care was primarily about meeting your own needs rather than those of a patient or carer.
- How might you have done things differently in order to meet the needs of the service user and your own needs?

For chaplains
- What are the theological issues that Edith needs to address to improve her practice and to look after her own well-being?
- Theologically, what informs how you seek to achieve balance in your work between being with and supporting others, and time away to perform other tasks at work or have time off?

As human beings and healthcare professionals all of us want to be needed and valued. If we are honest, part of our motivation for working in healthcare is that our vocational role helps to fulfil such needs. This is normal and, if acknowledged, perfectly healthy. However, we may establish particular patterns of behaviour in our professional roles informed by needs within us (like Edith) which, if unrecognised and not owned, may in the long term harm us and be detrimental to patient care, and perhaps to multi-disciplinary teamwork. When, with the help of supportive others, the link between our ways of working and behaving and our inner needs can be made, steps can then be taken to address those needs in a more helpful way.

DEALING WITH EXISTENTIAL QUESTIONS

'Why' is a small word, but a hugely perplexing and challenging question. Trying to respond appropriately to the existential wrestling of service users is an experience not unfamiliar to healthcare practitioners, whatever the context or sector in which we work. As people struggle to come to terms with diagnoses, debilitating illness or injury, or to adjust to loss or bereavement, they commonly verbalise questions such as:
- Why me?
- What have I done to deserve this?
- How can this happen to my loved one when he has lived a good life?
- How can there be a God?

Seeking answers to such existential questions which are provoked by human suffering, often suffering that is understood or perceived to be undeserved, is a lifelong quest. How best can we support those who seek meaning and understanding at times of tragedy, uncertainty and loss?

Case Scenario 8.4 and Reflective Activity 8.7 will help you to engage with responding to distress and existential questions.

CASE SCENARIO 8.4

Sharon had lived with manic depression for ten years. She was diagnosed two years after she married Gordon. Together with their two children, Lisa, aged six, and Andrew, aged four, they coped as best they could. They all had a very good relationship with Jim, Sharon's community psychiatric nurse. Unfortunately, while recovering from a period of deep and debilitating depression that required hospitalisation, Sharon hung herself in the family's garage. Gordon found his wife when he came home from shopping, but was unsuccessful in trying to resuscitate her with a neighbour. The children were with their grandparents at the time.

A month after the funeral, Jim called in to see Gordon in the family home. He had visited two weeks previously, but Gordon was busy with the children, so they had arranged a time when they could speak alone together. After Gordon had made a cup of tea, Jim asked specifically how he was.

Gordon broke down in tears and, between sobs, said:
'Why? Why us?
Why now? The kids are only young ... they need a mum.
It's not fair ... that bloody disease!'

Reflective Activity 8.7

What feelings may Gordon be experiencing?
What issues may underlie such feelings?
If you were Jim, how would you respond?
What would you say, or not say?
What would you do?

What is important to Gordon is not the answer to his questions right now, but the opportunity to vent his feelings – to be who he really is at that moment in time and express himself as he really needs to.

Henri Nouwen, cited by Salt, describes beautifully the kind of person Gordon might wish to have supporting him at such a traumatic time:[6]

> When we honestly ask ourselves which persons in our lives mean the most to us, we often find it is those who instead of giving advice, solutions or cures, have chosen instead to share our pain. The friend who can be silent with us in an hour of grief, who can tolerate not knowing, not curing, not healing, and face with us the reality of our powerlessness is the friend that cares.

It is hard to stay with someone and not have the answers or be able to do something to alleviate or take away such pain. However, if we are able to stay with them for a while, if this is what they want, such a gesture says 'You are not alone – I care and you matter.' The significance of a practitioner's willingness to be with another in their distress and confusion, along with the manner in which we wait with or accompany them, can never be underestimated. Our presence and our way of being and relating are seldom forgotten, whereas our words or task-related actions often are.[7]

With regard to Case Scenario 8.4, Gordon, quite naturally, will have myriad feelings within him, some of which may have built up over years and some of which are directly related to recent events. Jim is obviously someone Gordon feels safe with and with whom he feels he can be open and vulnerable. At an appropriate moment, Jim enquires about him specifically, and not the children (as most of his family and friends have been doing). As he supports Gordon in his distress, Jim actually needs to say very little. Rather, he needs to convey by his way of being and relating that he is willing to stay with Gordon as he expresses his deeply felt emotion, and that he is not judging Gordon or making him feel weak or silly at a time of great vulnerability. Jim might gently say 'I don't know' or 'I wonder why, too.' He might crouch down beside Gordon if Gordon is sitting with his head in his hands. He might perhaps put his hand on Gordon's shoulder or arm, or put his arm around the back of Gordon's chair or indeed around his shoulder, or give him a hug.

Reflective Activity 8.8 will help you to explore your attitudes to touch as part of spiritual care in clinical practice.

Reflective Activity 8.8

In Case Scenario 8.4, if you were Jim how would you feel about touching Gordon?
- What might touching Gordon on the arm or shoulder convey?
- Why might you touch Gordon, or why might you not touch him?
- If Gordon was a woman or an openly gay man, would that influence your decision as to whether to touch? What if Gordon was someone you found sexually attractive?
- Reflect on whether touching another person in order to indicate compassionate care as opposed to functional touch is part of your professional practice.
- Would you hug Gordon?
- Are there ever circumstances when you definitely would not hug a service user?
- What if Gordon had actively asked you for a hug in similar circumstances? How would you have reacted?

Touch can convey care, compassion, concern and empathy when words seem inadequate. Touch can also meet our need to do something when we feel helpless, or it can be a means by which we seek to soothe someone and stop them crying – the action therefore meeting our need, not that of the other person.

TOUCH AS PART OF SPIRITUAL CARE

To touch another person is risky, for touch is physical, bodily, and thus sexual. Our sexuality is not just the genital expression of our desires, nor is it simply related to orientation. We are sexual beings because we inhabit physical bodies – we are embodied beings. How we relate to others, male and female, old and young, involves our physical or sexual selves through gesture, posture and touch, as well as through words and silence. Touch is risky, therefore, because it involves offering ourselves, or at least part of ourselves, to others, and this gesture of self can either be accepted and appreciated or rejected. The rejection of our touch can hurt because the physical aspect of ourselves is a big part of who we are as people. It can be perceived as rejection of all of our care and best intentions. Therefore, we sometimes hold back and don't risk touching even when we discern that touch might be appropriate and appreciated. However, to touch another person when this is not wanted, even with the best of intentions, can be perceived as a threat or as a reminder of deeper hurts. Hence, as with all aspects of healthcare, those with whom we work should always feel that they have a choice – to accept or refuse the offer of compassionate touch without being made to feel guilty either way.

There are times when we offer touch as a means of comfort and support and get it wrong. We will misread cues or be less than discerning and people will withdraw their hand from ours or wince at a gently placed hand on a forearm or shoulder. However, with reflection on our practice and the courage to learn from our mistakes, hopefully we shall keep on daring to touch, as and when we feel that it is appropriate and permission is granted. For when patients and their loved ones are most vulnerable, gentle and discerning touch is a highly meaningful way to convey genuine care, love and compassion, especially when words are insufficient.

LISTENING TO STORIES AS SPIRITUAL CARE

In being present, in our attentiveness to the moment and in the warmth and acceptance that we may convey, service users often find encouragement not just to share their feelings, but to tell their stories. In the telling of their stories, sometimes repeatedly, patients and relatives may not only put their present situation into a broader perspective, but they may also be able to re-interpret or re-frame what has happened in a different way. In doing so, some may find meaning and fragments of understanding in their experiences; others will not, and will continue to seek these in their own way. Storytelling, in the context of bereavement, is not only about meaning making, but also affords the opportunity to create and shape memories.[8,9]

Disenfranchised grief – for example, following suicide, stillbirth or murder (open discussion of which is often not considered socially acceptable) – may mean that there are few if any opportunities for bereaved people to talk about their deceased loved one and share stories about their life together. This is because other family members, friends and neighbours, as well as the bereaved person him- or herself, may be reticent about initiating such conversations.[10] In these cases a healthcare professional may well have a key role in facilitating such conversations.

Reflective Activity 8.9 invites you to explore the idea of facilitating storytelling.

Reflective Activity 8.9

Returning to Case Scenario 8.4:
- Once Gordon's sobbing has stopped and he has calmed down a little, if you were Jim how would you encourage him to tell his story and the story of his life together with Sharon?
  - What sort of prompts might you use?
- What issues might it be helpful to explore with Gordon? Perhaps you might want to think again about what Gordon might be feeling (*see* Reflective Activity 8.7).

Often, in such situations, reflecting back a short statement made by the service user, or a feeling that has been picked up (e.g. 'It is so unfair' or 'No wonder you are angry') will facilitate storytelling which requires the listener to say very little indeed as a whole lot of related issues and feelings may be shared. Other helpful prompts in bereavement situations involve asking about the deceased and their life with the bereaved. For example, if you were Jim you could ask Gordon what Sharon was like when she was well (Jim only knew her as a patient with manic depression), or how they first met. In Gordon's case, particular issues of anger, guilt and shame, and dealing with the internal images that he carries of finding Sharon hanging in their garage, may need to be explored. This may be beyond your limitations, both professionally and personally, and therefore it is important to reflect about an appropriate individual to whom you might refer Gordon.

For more detailed information on specifically supporting suicide survivors see, for example, *Grief Counselling and Grief Therapy* by Worden.[11]

RITUAL AS PART OF SPIRITUAL CARE

Healthcare is infused with ritual. Multi-disciplinary meetings and handovers within professional groups are good examples of this. Stories are shared, care plans emerge, actions are agreed, interactions are invested in, and meaning and purpose are given to the shift, the day or the week. Routine is also part and parcel of what we construct individually and collectively to give shape to our work and to enable the health service to function. Patients are woken, breakfast is taken, toileting and washing occur and ward rounds take place in the same order on most days, enabling a ward community to orientate itself and run reasonably efficiently. What is the difference between ritual and routine? Ritual is action that is invested with significant meaning by those who are participating in it. 'A routine can become a ritual if it transforms an instrumental and perfunctory act into a symbolically charged experience that may be repeated in memory.'[12] For example, changing the nappy of your baby and washing and dressing her is a routine task. However, if your baby is stillborn and you do this activity only once, as you simultaneously say hello and goodbye, it becomes infused with meaning and most certainly becomes a ritual.

Ritual is important in spiritual care when words are insufficient and a change or transition needs to be marked. It can be a private act or a communal activity that binds and holds people together.

At its best, ritual evolves out of story and situation and is not alien or forced on to either. Ritual needs to involve participative actions, language that all can understand, and silence which can be shared. Yet it points to or represents something more which can potentially be transformative. Rituals can be repeated and woven into the regular pattern of life, like religious worship, or they can be one-off events. In healthcare, they are best co-created by the practitioner and service user together, informed by the stories that have been told and heard and the resources and knowledge that each brings to the relationship.

The continuation of Case Scenario 8.4 involving Gordon and Jim will help healthcare workers from any discipline to reflect on the possible therapeutic use of ritual in the delivery of spiritual care.

CASE SCENARIO 8.4 CONTINUED

As Gordon begins to share with Jim the story of life together with Sharon, including the shared joys as well as great challenges and frustrations, he talks of how their family home feels as if it has become dominated by great sadness and the violence of the means of her death. Gordon feels that all the happy and special times, especially those shared in the house with their children, have been tarnished by events of the past few weeks. He also regrets listening to the strong advice given by members of the family that Lisa and Andrew should not attend Sharon's funeral and now wonders if they should have included the children more in the ritual marking of Sharon's life as well as her tragic death.

Reflective Activity 8.10

For all healthcare practitioners
- If you were Jim, what might you suggest as a means of helping Gordon to deal with his concerns?
- How do you think the construction and sharing in an appropriate ritual with Gordon and his children (and anyone else whom he feels that he wants to include) might help?

(continued)

> **For chaplains**
>
> Jim has contacted you with regard to his conversation with Gordon.
> * Reflect on some basic principles and theological themes that will inform how you might approach constructing such a ritual and who you might involve in its construction and performance. For example, whose ritual is it, what is your role, and what is the purpose of such a ritual?
> * How would you go about constructing a ritual in this case?
> * What might the ritual involve? (Think, for example, about ritual action, symbols, images, words and music.)
> * What resources do you have that you can offer to Gordon and any others involved to help them to make informed choices?

Ritual that meets real rather than assumed spiritual need not only develops out of the stories shared by practitioner and service user(s), but should also be co-constructed. By sharing information, relevant resources and cultural norms (examples of what others have done in similar circumstances, as in Case Scenario 8.1), a practitioner enables patients and carers to make informed choices, regain some control and have ownership of the ritual (where this is wanted). Ritual enables the enactment and affirmation of relationships, gives space for wrestling and searching, creates significant memories and, in and of itself, can give meaning and orientation at a time which may otherwise be devoid of both.

A concluding complex case scenario is now offered to close this chapter. Although it includes echoes of Gordon and Sharon's story, it occurs in a different context and involves engaging with some contrasting spiritual issues and possible responses.

CASE SCENARIO 8.5

Eva is a 16-year-old girl who has been knocked down in the street while on holiday with her father Bill, her best friend Liz, and her younger brother Simon. All three were with her at the time of the incident. On arrival at the Accident and Emergency department of the local hospital the staff urgently work on Eva while her family and Liz are shown into the family room.

Unfortunately, nothing can be done for Eva and she is pronounced dead soon after arrival. Bill, who is a member of the choir in his local church, asks for a chaplain to come and be with him and Liz and Simon while they wait. The chaplain barely has a chance to introduce herself when a doctor and nurse who have been involved in Eva's care arrive to tell her family and Liz that she has died.

Reflective Activity 8.11 asks you to reflect not only on this case scenario but also on your own experience of working in similar situations, and how you dealt with them.

Reflective Activity 8.11

For all healthcare practitioners

- How might the doctor and nurse involved be feeling at this moment and after they have been with this family?
- What issues might contribute to those feelings?
- Where might the Accident and Emergency doctor and nurse take their feelings and the issues associated with those feelings?
- What might you do with your feelings and the thoughts provoked by such an experience?
- What is the role of the chaplain in such a scenario?

For chaplains

- How might you feel in such a situation?
- What issues might contribute to those feelings?
- What is your role at this point?
- How would you relate to the family and to the doctor and nurse?
- What would you say and do at this point?

Case Scenario 8.5 now continues to unfold, and you are encouraged to explore how you respond to the meaning, or sheer senselessness, that others find in tragic circumstances (note that Reflective Activity 8.2 looked at our response to service users' different coping mechanisms in response to illness or loss).

CASE SCENARIO 8.5 CONTINUED

Bill, Liz and Simon all react differently after they hear the terrible news. Bill, a widower, keeps repeating 'I can't believe it, I can't believe it' and puts his head in his hands and weeps. Simon, aged nine, looks totally bewildered and goes to cuddle and comfort his dad. Liz sits almost detached from what is going on and shrugs off the notion of any form of physical comforting from the nurse who kneels beside her and tries to take her hand. After a few minutes the doctor and nurse withdraw, saying that the chaplain can come and get one of them if there is anything else that the family wants to know or ask. The chaplain says very little, but puts her arm around Bill as he starts to sob again. He in turn cuddles Simon. Liz sits at the opposite side of the room. Gradually Bill's crying subsides and the room quietens, and then out of the silence Liz spits at the chaplain 'How can you sit here, you and your bloody God? How can there be a God to let this happen?' Bill looks aghast, and says to her 'Liz, God obviously needed Eva. He needed Eva to keep her mum company.'

Reflective Activity 8.12

- How would you react to these statements made by Liz and Bill?
- Which of the statements, if any, could you relate to? Why?
- How would you respond, in your professional role, in this situation?

It not just as healthcare professionals that we have to deal with others' beliefs and attempts at meaning making – they touch our interpretation and understanding of our personal experiences and beliefs, too. What do we each do with this? How do you process the impact of spiritual issues that you have to deal with at work as they affect your own spirituality?

The final two parts of Case Scenario 8.5 are primarily intended for chaplains, but other healthcare professionals will find it worth engaging with them, as they will also help you to reflect further on your own beliefs about death and the possibility of an afterlife (and what form that may take). These issues are especially significant if you have to support others who may be wrestling with these end-of-life issues.

CASE SCENARIO 8.5 CONTINUED

After a while the nurse returns and asks if the family needs anything, and offers them the use of a phone, as well as a cup of tea. Bill phones his brother and Liz phones her mother. Later, the nurse asks whether anyone would like to see Eva, and explains that although her legs and chest have severe injuries, her face is relatively unscathed. Liz quickly nods and Bill indicates that he would like to see his daughter. Simon is not so sure. His dad gently encourages him, remembering how he wished that he had let Eva see her mother after her death (Simon was only a toddler). The nurse asks Simon if he would show her how Eva liked her hair done, as they are trying to brush it for her and they want to get it right. Simon nods and Bill asks the chaplain to accompany them.

On seeing his daughter, Bill begins to sob again and gives her a kiss. Liz also kisses her friend and accepts an arm round her shoulder from Bill. Simon, once he overcomes his initial wariness, is engrossed for a minute or two in showing the nurse how to arrange his big sister's hair. The nurse comments to Simon how beautiful his big sister is. Simon agrees and turns to the chaplain and asks 'Will she look like this in heaven? Will my mum be beautiful too?'

Reflective Activity 8.13

- How would you respond to Simon?
- What feelings and issues might arise for you, if you were involved in this scenario at this stage?
- What are your beliefs about an afterlife? Have they changed since you became involved in healthcare?

Part of the final case scenario involves a request for prayer – a religious ritual which is performed silently by many in healthcare every day, or on occasions is requested to be said by someone who is perceived to have religious authority.

CASE SCENARIO 8.5 CONTINUED

Around Eva, once their tears have subsided, Bill, Liz and Simon begin to talk a bit about her – how her appearance was important to her, her interest in dancing, music and boys, how she looked out for her brother and her dad as well as being a loyal yet stubborn friend. The chaplain gently facilitates this storytelling along with the nurse. After a few minutes Bill asks the chaplain to say a prayer.

This penultimate activity helps you to look at the significance of prayer in spiritual care. It will help you to reflect on its purpose and what prayers might involve and include.

Reflective Activity 8.14

For all healthcare practitioners
- Why might it be important to Bill that it is the chaplain who says the prayer, rather than anyone else involved?
- What might be the purpose of the prayer as perceived by Bill?

For chaplains
- How would you approach saying the prayer? What resources would you utilise?
- What would you include in the prayer?
- Would you use any ritual action in the prayer? For example, would you touch Eva or ask everyone around Eva to hold hands?
- How else might you care for those involved in this scenario, including yourself as chaplain?

SPIRITUAL CARE AS RESPECTFUL ABSENCE

Much has been written about the significance of an attentive reassuring presence in the provision of spiritual care. Being with others at a time of waiting and uncertainty or anxiety and distress can enable them to feel listened to and of value. Out of such relationships, spiritual needs can be assessed, information can be shared, informed choices and referrals can be made, and ritual can be constructed as appropriate. However, just as important after presence in spiritual care provision is respectful absence; this is necessary for both the service user and the practitioner (*see* Case Scenario 8.3). Patients and their loved ones require time alone in which to reflect on and process information and experiences, to consider options and make necessary decisions or practical arrangements. For healthcare workers, time away from caring is a necessity as it enables them to reflect on practice, to let go and to play. If practitioners do not discern and act upon the need to find a balance between being present and being absent in caring relationships where spiritual care is offered, especially in complex situations of need, they will sooner or later become drained and experience burnout.

Finally, Reflective Activity 8.15 will help you to consider the important issue of endings, whether permanent or temporary, to a therapeutic relationship in which spiritual care has been delivered.

Reflective Activity 8.15

- How would you approach taking your leave from the family in Case Scenario 8.5 once you feel that you have done all you can for them at this moment in time, or because it is the end of your shift?
- What would you say or do as an ending (to meet their needs and yours)?
- In similar circumstances, what cues or prompts (in others, in you and in the circumstances) do you look for to help you to discern that it is time to take your leave?

Responding to service users' spiritual needs potentially involves all healthcare staff, and ranges from treating them with dignity and respect to empowering informed choice in decision making and accompanying others at a most traumatic and vulnerable time. Chaplains, as specialist providers, are a resource that healthcare practitioners can utilise to help to meet the complex spiritual and religious needs of those in their care.

FURTHER READING

➤ Cobb M. *The Hospital Chaplain's Handbook*. Norwich: The Canterbury Press; 2005.
➤ Gilbert P. *Guidelines on Spirituality for Staff in Acute Care Services*. Leeds: Care Services Improvement Partnership; 2008.
➤ Grant E, Murray S, Kendall M *et al.* Spiritual issues and needs: perspectives from patients with advanced cancer and non-malignant disease: a qualitative study. *Palliative and Supportive Care* 2004; **2**: 371–8.
➤ Johnstone Taylor E. *What Do I Say? Talking with patients about spirituality*. Philadelphia, PA: Templeton Foundation Press; 2007.
➤ Koenig H. *Spirituality in Patient Care: why, how, when and what*, 2nd edn. Philadelphia, PA: Templeton Foundation Press; 2007.
➤ Orchard H (ed). *Spirituality in Health Care Contexts*. London: Jessica Kingsley Publishers; 2001.
➤ Smith H, Smith M. *Helping Others: being around, being there, being wise*. London: Jessica Kingsley Publishers; 2008.
➤ Stoter D. *Spiritual Aspects of Healthcare*, 2nd edn. Eugene, OR: Wipf and Stock Publishers; 2008.
➤ White G. *Talking about Spirituality in Healthcare Practice: a resource for the multi-disciplinary health care team*. London: Jessica Kingsley Publishers; 2006.
➤ Wright B. *Sudden Death: a research base for practice*. Philadelphia, PA: Churchill Livingstone; 1985.

REFERENCES

 1 Scottish Government. *The Healthcare Quality Strategy for NHS Scotland*. Edinburgh: Scottish Government; 2010. www.scotland.gov.uk (accessed January 2011).

 2 Quinlan J. *Journey Through Dying, Death and Bereavement*. Dublin: The Columba Press; 1989. p. 33.

 3 Galloway K. *Struggles to Love: the spirituality of the Beatitudes*. London: SPCK; 1994.

 4 MacDiarmid H. The two parents. In: Riach A, Grieve M (eds) *Hugh MacDiarmid: Selected Poetry*. Manchester: Carcanet Press Limited; 2004. p. 169.

 5 Hawkins P, Shohet R. *Supervision in the Helping Professions*. Milton Keynes: Open University Press; 2007.

 6 Salt S. Towards a definition of suffering. *European Journal of Palliative Care* 1997; **4:** 60.

 7 Kelly E. *Marking Short Lives: constructing and sharing rituals following pregnancy loss*. Oxford: Peter Lang; 2007.

 8 Anderson H, Foley E. *Mighty Stories, Dangerous Rituals*. San Francisco, CA: Jossey-Bass Inc., Publishers; 1998.

 9 Walter T. *On Bereavement: the culture of grief*. Buckingham: Open University Press; 1999.

10 Worden J. *Grief Counselling and Grief Therapy: a handbook for the mental health practitioner*, 3rd edn. New York: Springer Publishing Co.; 2002.

11 Worden J. *Grief Counselling and Grief Therapy: a handbook for the mental health practitioner*, op. cit.

12 Romanoff B, Thompson B. Meaning construction in palliative care: the use of narrative, ritual, and the expressive arts, *American Journal of Hospice and Palliative Care* 2006; **23:** 309–16.

CHAPTER 9

Ethics and values in spiritual care practice

INTRODUCTION

As has been previously explored, particularly in Chapter 8, the provision of spiritual care is not simply what is *done* to or with a service user, but *how* a practitioner relates and performs required tasks. This chapter seeks to help healthcare staff to reflect on their personal values and moral perspectives which influence both personal and communal practice. This moral dimension of our humanity significantly informs our identity – our sense of who we are. Our moral code shapes not only our contribution to decisions that are made in our workplace, but also our behaviour and our attitudes to others and their ethical perspectives. Former healthcare chaplain David Lyall suggests that there is no such thing as 'value-free' counselling.[1] The provision of other aspects of healthcare, including spiritual care and ethical decision making, is similarly value-laden.

Bioethics, for example, is not performed in a vacuum nor is it simply a science where guiding principles and rules can be applied to any situation to enable a decision to be made which is in a patient's best interests. Decision making in healthcare is an art performed by human beings, healthcare staff, patients and their carers, who all bring their own personal values, beliefs and opinions to any particular situation. Moreover, any ethical choice that is made has implications which potentially impinge on the personal and shared meanings, sense of fulfilment and worldviews of all those involved. That is to say, bioethical decision making creates potential spiritual need, even distress, in patients, their carers and healthcare staff.

The authors passionately believe that deepening self-awareness is a significant ongoing activity in the promotion of best practice in spiritual care delivery (*see also* Chapters 1 and 8) and also in bioethical decision making. Our unique moral framework, through which we interpret actions, but which also informs our opinions, judgements and way of being has evolved from our childhood onwards. It is continually being reshaped and remodelled as we reflect on experience and practice throughout our lives. The more aware we are of our own moral landscape, the better we can make room for, identify and hopefully respect another's. Key ethical principles which influence bioethical decision making and ways of relating in healthcare will be used as tools to help the reader to engage with their personal value base and moral frame of reference. These will include:

➤ autonomy
➤ beneficence
➤ non-maleficence
➤ justice.

In addition, the concept of virtue as a value which gives 'direction and substance to practice' will be explored.[2]

AUTONOMY

In ancient Greece, the term 'autonomy', *autonomia*, was used to describe the independence of city states which allowed them to determine their own laws free from outside interference. In contemporary society, autonomy is related to the freedom to think, decide and act independently without hindrance.[3] Within healthcare, autonomy is considered 'first among equals' as a guiding moral principle that informs practice and decision making.[4] In order to make autonomous choices, a person needs to be rational in their thinking, understand their situation, and not be coerced into making particular decisions.

Case Scenario 9.1 and Reflective Activity 9.1 will help you to explore something of your understanding of, and attitude towards, the concept of patient autonomy within healthcare. Bioethical decision making in the twenty-first century has become increasingly complex, and more than one guiding principle or influencing factor will need to be considered at any time. However, here we shall concentrate on the principle of autonomy.

CASE SCENARIO 9.1

Ms B, a 43-year-old professional woman, had a second haemorrhage in her upper spinal cord which left her permanently quadriplegic and dependent on artificial ventilation. Ms B went to great lengths to find out about her long-term prognosis. Due to her condition she felt that life would be intolerable due to a lack of control over her own body, and her dependence on others. As a consequence, she sought to have her ventilator switched off and to be allowed to die. The doctors involved in her care felt unable to carry out her wishes. However, the High Court ruled that she had 'the necessary mental capacity to give consent or to refuse life-sustaining medical treatment.'

Following this ruling, Ms B was taken off her ventilator and treated according to her wishes, including the prescription of medication to enable her to die peacefully.[5]

Reflective Activity 9.1

Reflecting on Case Scenario 9.1, you are now encouraged to consider what values and moral perspectives you might have brought (in relation to autonomy) to Ms B's care and the process of her decision making.

- How do you feel about the perspective of:
  - Ms B
  - the doctors
  - the court?
- If you were part of the multi-disciplinary team looking after Ms B, would you align yourself with Ms B or with the doctors?
- What informs your ethical stance on this? Consider:
  - your upbringing
  - your personal beliefs and worldview
  - your personal experience (including interaction with media, film and books)
  - your professional experience.
- Has engaging with this case scenario altered, or confirmed, any aspect of your understanding of the place of a patient's autonomy in the process of bioethical decision making?

The case of Ms B reveals that respecting another's autonomy can be problematic, especially if it requires the carrying out of actions which conflict with our understanding of beneficence and non-maleficence.

BENEFICENCE

Beneficence is the act of 'doing good'. For healthcare practitioners this means seeking what they consider best for a patient according to their clinical acumen, reflected experience and knowledge. In practice, this also means that *to do good* is also to seek *to do no harm*, which requires the following:

➤ **practitioner competence, capability and ongoing professional and personal development:** staff will need to have the knowledge and skills necessary to care for a conscious ventilated patient over a long period of time, as well as being able to keep her comfortable after extubation

➤ **respect for patient choice/autonomy:** in the case of Ms B, staff involved in her care will need to ensure they convey to her that they have heard and understood as best they can what her wishes are and the reasons behind them

➤ **good communication:** in the case of Ms B, staff will need to be able not only to communicate complex facts but also to convey empathy, warmth and a non-judgemental attitude in order to build up a trusting relationship in which challenging issues (for both the patient and staff members) would need to be explored.

Reflective Activity 9.2 will help you to engage with issues of beneficence, what the term means for you, and how beneficence can be constrained by the patient's wishes.

Reflective Activity 9.2

> From your personal life experience, consider the following questions:
> - What did 'doing good' mean when you were growing up?
> - Think of some examples of occasions when you were praised for doing good.
>
> Reflect again on Case Scenario 9.1 and the situation of Ms B.
> - What were the doctors' motives for not withdrawing life support initially?
> - For you, what would 'doing good' for Ms B involve? Consider the reasons why.

It can be difficult to separate out beneficence as a motivating factor for decision making from non-maleficence. Doing no harm may well have been the primary factor that the doctors considered when refusing at first to comply with Ms B's wishes. Or it may have been that switching off her ventilator was not perceived as doing good and acting in her best interests. Or possibly both of these factors were involved.

NON-MALEFICENCE

The concept of non-maleficence is demonstrated as part of the Hippocratic Oath, *primum non nocere* – 'First of all (at least) do no harm.' Doctors and other healthcare staff have a duty not to harm patients or expose them to risk of harm without clear justification.

Reflective Activity 9.3 will help you to reflect further on the principle of *primum non nocere* and how ethical principles inform our way of relating and caring.

Reflective Activity 9.3

> - If in Case Scenario 9.1 you were involved in Ms B's care as she was exploring her spiritual need for control, meaning and purpose in her life, how might the concept of non-maleficence influence your support of her?
> - If you morally disagreed with Ms B's desire to have her ventilator switched off, how might that affect the person-centred spiritual care you sought to offer?
> - Considering this dilemma, what would you do with any potential internal moral conflicts which may arise from your work in a healthcare setting?

Doing no harm (as with other guiding principles) in healthcare is not just related to physical care, but also underpins holistic, including spiritual, care.

It involves respect for the service user's beliefs, values and decisions. Therefore any attempt to coerce or persuade a patient to change their moral perspective or worldview is not only an abuse of power, but is also contrary to the principle of non-maleficence.

JUSTICE

In contemporary healthcare, consideration of the allocation of available resources has become an increasingly contentious issue. Financially, the public purse is finite, and how we as a society should decide what aspects of healthcare deserve continued, enhanced or reduced funding is a major challenge. Justice demands equity of access to appropriate care for patients in relation to their needs, whatever their socio-economic background.

Aristotle was a philosopher in ancient Greece who was a student of Plato and a teacher of Alexander the Great. For him, justice meant fair and proportionate treatment – equals should be treated equally, and unequals in proportion to relevant inequalities. For example, two people admitted through an Accident and Emergency department with leg fractures that require surgery but who are otherwise stable should be treated equally. However, if in the meantime a patient is admitted with life-threatening multiple injuries after a car crash, that person deserves immediate surgery and takes precedence in theatre over the other two waiting casualties.

Reflective Activity 9.4 is designed to help you to consider some issues relating to justice in healthcare, and to reflect on your attitudes in relation to equity of access to care.

Reflective Activity 9.4

In Case Scenario 9.1, caring for Ms B in an intensive-care unit will have cost thousands of pounds each week. While she remained ventilated, other critically ill patients could not have access to the intensive-care bed that she occupied and the related technology and care that she benefited from in that particular hospital location.
- Would you consider Ms B's care to be a significant drain on healthcare resources? If so, would you consider that this prevented others from accessing specialist care when she did not want to continue living?
- Had Ms B been a less well-informed, eloquent and determined individual, do you think her wishes would still have been fulfilled?
- If you think not, is this just?
- If you were involved in caring for Ms B, how might these issues have affected your attitude towards her and thus, even unconsciously, your support of her?

Our values and ethical perspectives influence not only how we act and our process of ethical decision making, but also how we relate to others.

VIRTUE

Plato was a philosopher and mathematician in ancient Greece, who founded the Academy in Athens, which was the first institute of higher learning in the Western world. Both he and Aristotle talked of virtue as that which enabled people to hold on to their integrity and character in the face of adversity and oppression.[6] In Latin, the word virtue is derived from *virtus*, meaning strength or the ability to accomplish. Thus:

> virtues are the qualities of the person that enable something to be brought into being, i.e. moral virtues enable moral meaning and purpose to be embodied. By extension they are the qualities that enable a spiritual ethos to be lived out in individual and corporate practice. Hence, we would normally refer to the virtues of the individual, but also it is possible to see the term in relation to a community or a group, i.e. describing a group as having integrity.[7]

Virtue is a key part of who we are as moral beings. It is a core part of our identity or our character, and as Robinson suggests it significantly shapes how we perceive groups or communities to behave or relate.[7]

Reflective Activity 9.5

> • Consider the doctors in Case Scenario 9.1 to be representative of the whole intensive-care multi-disciplinary team. From their moral stance and decision making, how might you describe this group of healthcare professionals?

Whether or not we agree with that particular healthcare team's collective moral perspective, they were courageous and acted with integrity and honesty. They had faith that their stance was appropriate even when their decision making was challenged and then overturned in the High Court (and given considerable public airing in the British media).

Plato postulated that as human beings we can intuitively recognise or know what is good and virtuous, but for Aristotle, virtue 'is a disposition a person has towards making good choices, and the way we learn to make good choices is through imitation.'[8] As children we learn through imitating the decision making and ways of relating of significant people and groups in our formative years to develop the habit of making good choices (or not). Jamison helpfully goes on to say:[8]

> Platonic contemplation involves knowing the good, the sense of knowing being like that of knowing a friend rather than knowing a fact. Aristotelian virtue involves doing good, as in living out the virtues.

Reflective Activity 9.6 will help you to explore how your moral character developed in your younger years, and what virtues you may possess that influence the therapeutic relationships which you form.

Reflective Activity 9.6

Re-read your response to Reflective Activity 9.1 and revisit your thoughts as an introduction to this next task.
- Who were the key people, groups and communities in your upbringing whose behaviour, choices and ways of relating you imitated?
- Would you consider that such 'imitating' was conscious or unconscious, or a combination of both?
- What was it about them that you found life-affirming or that you admired?
- How would you describe their traits, characteristics or principles?
- To what extent do you find that you embody or live out these traits in your role as a healthcare professional?

Robinson suggests that virtues are transmitted through the stories we hear, and are modelled in significant relationships.[9] In our therapeutic relationships with others we may embody good and make good choices, but potentially we can learn more of what is good as it is experienced in relationship with service users. Our moral character grows and develops through a process of habituation (or impersonating), embodying, engagement with others (practice) and reflection. Like our spiritual care provision, that which informs our behaviour and decision making is refined and re-shaped through reflective practice.

Robinson names the following virtues which inform and may be developed through spiritual care and reflective practice:
➤ integrity
➤ courage
➤ patience
➤ empathy
➤ humility
➤ honesty
➤ faith – not necessarily a religious faith but, for example, faith in self or others
➤ temperance – self-control, sense of balance
➤ hope
➤ *phronesis* (practical wisdom) – reflected experience and an ability to apply this with discernment in different contexts while being person-centred.

AGAPE

Agape is the Greek word for unconditional love, and this concept is central to the Judaeo-Christian tradition. However, it also resonates with the moral philosophy of other faith communities and belief groups. In addition, it is the vocational *raison d'être* of many practitioners who have no religious affiliation. However, love is not a word which is often made explicit in twenty-first-century healthcare. We may consider love to be an aspect of all the virtues listed above or, like Robinson, we may feel that it is the underlying basis of all healthcare activity and decision making.[10] Guiding principles and virtues may be felt to be complementary in helping healthcare practitioners to care ethically for service users, but love underpins both. Love demands care for all, and is the motivation to respond to those in need. It is necessary, therefore, to recapture the meaning, importance and expression of *agape*, such that we are not frightened of it or embarrassed by it in the delivery of high-quality holistic healthcare.

CHAPLAIN OR SPIRITUAL CARE PROFESSIONAL

Case Scenario 9.2 and Reflective Activities 9.7 and 9.8 will help chaplains in particular to reflect on the values and virtues that shape our practice. Specifically, engaging with this complex case scenario will challenge specialist spiritual care practitioners to explore the relationship between *agape* and personal virtues and values.

CASE SCENARIO 9.2

Bill and Moira are a married couple in their early forties with three school-age children. Unexpectedly, Moira has become pregnant again while Bill is on the waiting list for a vasectomy. They both have challenging but fulfilling jobs. Moira and the three children are active in their local church and various affiliated organisations. Bill attends worship occasionally. After various tests, at 18 weeks of pregnancy Moira and Bill are told that their baby has Down's syndrome. They had just begun to get their heads round being pregnant again, and now they are devastated. They wrestle at length with regard to what action to take, as their consultant obstetrician has raised the possibility of a termination. Their local minister is very helpful in supporting them as they express their feelings and fears and explore possible options and outcomes. During such discussions it emerges that their marriage has been going through a difficult period, and in the past Bill has struggled with bouts of depression, one episode being linked to the birth of their third child. They are also aware of a couple in their neighbourhood who are in their late seventies, whose daughter also has Down's syndrome and still lives with her parents.

In the end, at 22 weeks into the pregnancy, Moira and Bill opt for a termination. During Moira's induced labour they ask to see the on-call chaplain. They would like the chaplain to baptise their baby when he is born. All three of their other children have been baptised. Moira and Bill had called their own minister before coming into hospital, but he was unable to respond.

Reflective Activity 9.7 will help you to explore your attitudes towards and feelings about this request.

Reflective Activity 9.7

Reflecting on Case Scenario 9.2, consider the following:
- What would your personal moral perspective be with regard to such a situation? What informs that perspective?
- Might there be a theological perspective which should be considered?
- How would you deal professionally with Bill and Moira's request?
- Would this be in conflict with any of the four guiding principles that were considered earlier in the chapter?
- How would you deal with any inner moral dilemmas or tensions relating to responding to Bill and Moira's request?

There are times when our personal moral opinion may conflict with what we are asked to do in our professional role in seeking to deliver person-centred care. Moreover, some ethical values in healthcare may be in conflict not only with our own moral viewpoint but also with the beliefs and values of the faith community or belief group of which we are part.

CASE SCENARIO 9.2 CONTINUED

The on-call chaplain spent a long time listening to Bill and Moira's story and to their wishes. Gently she acknowledged the undoubted complexity, pain, guilt and loss involved. She went on to explain that members of their chaplaincy team did not baptise babies in this situation, but that she would be very happy to come and bless their baby when he was born, to help 'mark his unique and significant place in their family and God's family.' She also explained that, should they wish, the hospital would help them to organise a funeral for their baby, and the chaplaincy team were there to support them if required. This was another ritual which might help them to formally mark the importance of their baby's life and death and express their loss. Bill and Moira were happy with the idea of a blessing, and said that they would be keen to talk further about a funeral after the birth.

Baby Robert was born several hours later, and the chaplain responded immediately to the call from the labour suite. When the chaplain arrived Moira was holding her baby and Susan the midwife was listening to his heart. Moira said 'Robert's still alive. Will you baptise him?'

Reflective Activity 9.8

Following the development in Case Scenario 9.2:
- How would you respond to Moira's request? *'Robert's still alive. Will you baptise him?'* Think through your reasoning for your decision.
- How might engagement with this case scenario inform your future practice?

Wells and Quash argue that ethics is not so much about making good decisions as making good people.[11] The formation and re-formation of character is what is central to making decisions that not only have service users' best interests at heart and seek to do them no harm, but also enable that which is most loving. This includes wrestling with and responding to complex situations which we may never have faced before. Such character is formed not only by habit, repeatedly imitating and performing good practice, but by reflection on such practice and putting such learning into future practice. The art of spiritual care involves therapeutic use of self, including our moral character, which enables us through ongoing reflection to practise ethically and to keep learning about and developing our values base.

FURTHER READING

➤ Farvis R. Ethical considerations in spiritual care. *International Journal of Palliative Nursing* 2005; **11**: 189.

➤ Lammers S, Verhey A (eds). *On Moral Medicine: theological perspectives in medical ethics*, 2nd edn. Grand Rapids, MI: Wm. B. Eerdmans Publishing Co.; 1998.

➤ Messer N (ed.). *Theological Issues in Bioethics: an introduction with readings*. London: Darton, Longman and Todd; 2002.

➤ Verhey A. *Reading the Bible in the Strange World of Medicine*. Grand Rapids, MI: Wm. B. Eerdmans Publishing Co.; 2003.

REFERENCES

1 Lyall D. *Integrity of Pastoral Care*. London: SPCK; 2001.
2 Graham E. *Transforming Theology in an Age of Uncertainty*. Eugene, OR: Wipf and Stock Publishers; 2002.
3 Gillon R. *Philosophical Medical Ethics*. Chichester: John Wiley & Sons; 2003.
4 Gillon R. Ethics needs principles – four can encompass the rest – and respect for autonomy should be 'first among equals.' *Journal of Medical Ethics* 2003; **29**: 307–12.
5 Keown J. The case of Ms B: suicide's slippery slope? *Journal of Medical Ethics* 2002; **28**: 238–9.
6 Wells S, Quash B. *Introducing Christian Ethics*. Chichester: Wiley-Blackwell; 2010.
7 Robinson S. *Spirituality, Ethics and Care*. London: Jessica Kingsley Publishers; 2008. p. 113.
8 Jamison C. *Finding Happiness: monastic steps for a fulfilling life*. London: Phoenix; 2009. pp. 20–23.
9 Robinson S. *Spirituality, Ethics and Care*. London: Jessica Kingsley Publishers; 2008.
10 Robinson S. *Spirituality, Ethics and Care*, op. cit.
11 Wells S, Quash B. *Introducing Christian Ethics*. op. cit.

CHAPTER 10

Loss, grief and bereavement

INTRODUCTION

It is important to understand at the beginning of any exploration of loss that the issues are not confined to bereavement. Loss is about much more than death and dying. It touches all aspects of our living, and is an aspect of our humanity which we face on a regular basis in our personal lives and professional practice. It is true, of course, that the healthcare context inevitably involves facing the reality of dying and death, and, as a consequence, having to respond to those who are bereaved by the loss of a loved one, either suddenly or following a period of protracted illness. However, in all aspects of healthcare, patients themselves experience a multitude of losses – physical, psychological and social – all of which can and do contribute to spiritual distress.

This chapter will guide us through a progressive approach to loss, grief and bereavement, beginning with our personal experiences and understanding of loss, and then moving on to consider our professional practice in supporting patients and their family carers in their loss, grief and bereavement.

UNDERSTANDING LOSS

As with our understanding of spirituality, faith, belief and culture which has already been explored in previous chapters, self-awareness is the starting point for understanding loss. Reflective Activities 10.1, 10.2 and 10.3 lead us to explore our personal experiences of loss, guide us through the feelings and emotions that arise, and then invite us to consider how this understanding might inform our professional practice.

Reflective Activity 10.1

> Think of a time when you lost something that was important to you. Don't use a bereavement (i.e. the loss of a person), but concentrate on the loss of an object (e.g. a purse, keys, jacket, etc.). Go over the experience in your mind, and create a picture of the event. Think about the following:
> - What did you lose?

(continued)

- Where did this happen?
- What was going on around you at the time?
- What was the context of the loss?
- How important was the item that you lost?

You might want to write this down for future reference.

With this picture of a loss in your mind, Reflective Activity 10.2 will guide you to think through the impact of the loss.

Reflective Activity 10.2

Using your picture of the loss from Reflective Activity 10.1, try to recall the implications of the loss for you, and the circumstances that it created.
- What effect did the loss have on your plans?
- How important was the event to you?
- Who else became involved in the 'searching' process, and who was affected by the loss in addition to yourself?
- What other losses became connected with this loss? For example, if you lost your passport, did you also lose your flight, or your holiday, or your planned meeting, or the respect of your colleagues?

Again, you might find it helpful to write this down.

Our experiences of one loss will directly relate to the event in question, and may be common to all our experiences of loss. However, there are often also unique features personal to you – only you can decide on the importance of the loss. Reflective Activity 10.3 will take this same picture and now add the emotions that we experience in loss.

Reflective Activity 10.3

Using the story of your loss and the events that surrounded it, try to recall the feelings that this loss and its allied events caused in you. The list might include:
- confusion
- anger with yourself or other people
- embarrassment
- self-loathing
- feeling out of control
- despair
- frustration
- bewilderment.

The emotions that we feel are often strong ones which we are normally uncomfortable about showing, such as anger. It is normal when remembering such losses to feel the same emotions again, and this demonstrates the profound and lasting impact that loss can have on us. The feelings that losses generate are not confined to the time of each loss, but can be felt deeply when such a loss is recalled at a much later date, or when life events contrive to remind us of the pain and effect of a loss in the past.

Whether our story of loss is about car keys or travel instructions, a phone number or an address, a wedding ring or a credit card, we all know what it is to experience loss. Dealing with loss is integral to our experience of living. Exploring our losses demonstrates that loss is not a single event. It affects other aspects of our lives, and creates other (sometimes more difficult) losses which also have to be faced. The loss of the car keys, for example, might be stressful enough in itself, but if that loss means that you will be late picking up the children from school or will miss the time for your job interview, it will become even more significant. These losses may be compounded further when we consider the loss of 'calmness' (and, as a result, the loss of good driving skills) to be faced, and, at the end of it all, perhaps the loss of the job that we had hoped for.

Remembering loss also helps us recall the feelings that loss creates in us. These are feelings which are common to us all, and which are normal responses to the events that affect us. We know what they are about and, difficult though they are to process, we know that they are an expected response, in their varying degrees, to the events which we have to face.

If, in addition, our stories of loss are shared, we shall find that the reactions of others to our feelings are borne out of a empathy for our circumstances which comes from their own experiences. Likewise, the knowledge of our own feelings will lead us to understand what is being shared with and expressed to us. With this in mind, we begin to realise that our loss, the effect of it and the feelings that it generates are not only empathised with and understood by others out of their own experiences of loss, but also create mutuality with others when we have the opportunity to share our story with them.

Having explored our own experiences and understanding of loss, we shall now move on to look at the reactions that we see and experience in others during their experiences of loss, and we shall go deeper into this topic in order to explore our reactions to loss, known as grief.

UNDERSTANDING GRIEF AND BEREAVEMENT

Major losses are among the most spiritually destabilising circumstances that ever have to be faced in life. The effects of loss, and the trauma that surrounds dealing with it, go to the core of our spirituality, and raise profound questions about our meaning, purpose, worth, value, fulfilment, hope, and life progression.

Case Scenario 10.1 and Reflective Activity 10.4 introduce the impact that loss can have on individuals, and the nature of and reactions that commonly occur in grief.

CASE SCENARIO 10.1

Michael is a 32-year-old fireman who also plays semi-professional Rugby League. He is married to Alicia, and they have two young children, Aiden who is 7, and Jennifer who is 3. Alicia is 5 months pregnant with a third child. Michael has lost the use of both legs, one amputated below the knee and the other from the top of his thigh, as a result of a building collapsing on him during a major fire. He has been retired from the fire service on medical grounds, and is no longer able to play rugby. He is struggling with rehabilitation and adapting to the use of artificial limbs. During one particularly taxing session with his physiotherapist, he breaks down and confides, 'As if the loss of my legs wasn't bad enough. It's all the other bloody losses that go along with it that's so hard to bear. … Life's got bugger all to offer me anymore.'

Reflective Activity 10.4

Reflecting on Case Scenario 10.1 and from your own experience, consider the issues that are raised for Michael. Remember that losses can be physical, psychological, social and spiritual.
- What losses might Michael be experiencing?
- What are the feelings raised by these losses?
- What impact are these losses having on Michael's spirituality?

In recognising Michael's distress and using the strategies explored in Chapter 3 on dealing with difficult questions and strong emotion, how would you respond to his statement *'As if the loss of my legs wasn't bad enough. It's all the other bloody losses that go along with it that's so hard to bear. … Life's got bugger all to offer me anymore.'*

It is not surprising that coming to terms and living with loss takes a person into the depths of spiritual searching. An overwhelming hopelessness may prevail, bringing with it profound questions about the purpose of living, possible suicidal thoughts arising out of an immense despair, and, in specific cases, attempted or actual suicide itself.

The effects of loss in all of its manifestations on an individual's spirituality should not be underestimated. Consequently there has to be an understanding of the nature of loss and its destabilising effects before we begin to offer supportive responses to the patient's grief.

As healthcare professionals we are regularly challenged in our responses to loss, dealing as we do with breaking bad news, end-of-life care, grieving families and, where we have a particular interest, involvement with bereavement support. While those involved with such issues will inevitably draw on their resources of professional skills (e.g. good communication skills, therapeutic touch, good eye contact, empathy) to offer support and alleviate distress, there are few healthcare professionals who are specifically trained in loss and grief, and fewer still who will be able to relate such aspects to a spiritual destabilisation. It is therefore important to understand the territory of grief work, and past and present theories of loss and grief, in order to identify, assess and offer support to those experiencing spiritual distress.

Theories and models of loss, grief and bereavement

While the expectation is that the reader will explore for him- or herself the grief theories appropriate to his or her own line of research or study, it is worthwhile outlining the main theoretical frameworks at this stage. This will illustrate not only how theories have altered over the generations, but also that our understanding of loss has, to a large degree, 'settled down' into theories which are more flexible and accommodating of differences, and which are not tied to the more rigid 'linear theories' of earlier thought processes.

In the early part of the twentieth century, Sigmund Freud defined grief as a set of experiences which would usually follow a predictable course.[1] The human condition being what it is, he argued, means that there will be common responses in the human psyche to common events. The processes of grief could be predicted as 'normal'.

In the early 1960s, Erich Lindemann studied acute grief reactions experienced by individuals bereaved by natural causes, disasters and wars. Based on his observations, he was a pioneer in differentiating between normal and abnormal reactions to loss.[2] Clinical guidelines for the identification of abnormal grief reactions were a product of Lindemann's work.

The Kübler-Ross model was first introduced in 1969.[3] It describes a process by which people deal with grief and tragedy, which consists of five discrete stages, namely denial, anger, bargaining, depression and acceptance. Kübler-Ross originally applied these stages to people suffering from terminal illness, and later to those experiencing any form of catastrophic personal loss, including loss of job, loss of income, loss of freedom, divorce, drug addiction, the onset of a disease or chronic illness, an infertility diagnosis, and many tragedies and disasters. The five stages are not progressive, nor will they all be experienced by every patient.

John Bowlby was the first grief theorist to base his conclusions on empirical evidence.[4-6] The publication of his trilogy of books outlined the 'attachment theory', which identified how the circumstances surrounding the death of a loved one affected the characteristics, intensity and progress of the grieving process. According to Bowlby, only when the various phases of loss – from shock to disorganisation – have been successfully completed can a bereaved person, to a greater or lesser degree, begin a process of reorganisation and stabilisation.

Colin Murray Parkes was a former student of Bowlby, and after conducting bereavement research in Europe and the USA, he created a model of grief as a series of shifting pictures, one of which would be clearly evident for a time and would then fade while another one took precedence.[7] He postulated that the fact that the pictures of grief were not constant could begin to explain why grief was not experienced uniformly.

William Worden extended bereavement theory by presenting in his 1992 research and its revisions a unique critique of the 'mourning process.' This outlined what he defined as the four different 'tasks of mourning', namely accepting the reality of the loss, working through the pain of grief, adjusting to an environment in which the deceased is missing, and emotionally relocating the deceased and moving on with life. Worden was one of the first grief theorists to identify spiritual distress as a facet of loss.[8]

Dennis Klass, Phyllis Silverman and Steven Nickman published the theory of 'continuing bonds' in 1996.[9] Their studies showed that bereaved young people made an effort to reach out for a connection to the dead parent, and maintained their attachment in different ways. The 'continuing bonds' theory gained further acceptance as it began to be applied to other aspects of relational loss, such as the loss of a partner or a sibling.[10]

Tony Walter is another whose work provides a contrast to the more traditional 'stage' models of grieving. In *On Bereavement: the Culture of Grief*, Walter challenges the idea that all mourners need and want to 'let go' and 'move on'. He argues that many people maintain a healthy bond with their dead indefinitely, even while forging new social ties, and he explores how our cultural understanding has a huge impact upon the way in which we grieve.[11]

Margaret Stroebe and Henk Schut, both psychologists, postulated their 'dual process model' in 1999, depicting grief as an oscillatory process in which a bereaved individual alternately experiences and avoids the pain of grief during the same period of time, rather than in a linear fashion in which one stage has to end before another begins.[12]

An exploration of grief theories as they have unfolded over the past 100 years identifies the destabilising aspects of reactions to loss, and therefore the spiritual issues which arise. Understood through the 'linear' theories of the grief process (i.e. moving through stages until a resolution of the issues has been reached), as well as the 'adjustment' theories, such as those which explore 'continuing bonds' or a 'dual process', there will inevitably be questions which arise, such as 'Will I make it?', 'How can I survive this?', 'Will I ever get to a stage when I can live again?', 'Why is the grief journey so exhausting?', 'When will I feel stable again?' and 'How can I build a bond with a dead person into the rest of my living?' Such questions are profoundly spiritual in nature, and need to be understood in the same framework as other manifestations of spiritual distress.

DIFFERENT KINDS OF LOSS

As we have indicated above, bereavement is of course only one manifestation of loss. Issues that arise in other losses are exhibited in similar ways to those which are manifested in bereavement. There are multiple losses which are experienced by both patients and carers, all of which have a spiritual underpinning in aspects of meaning, purpose, fulfilment and hope.

Reflective Activity 10.5 will help us to develop our understanding of loss, grief and bereavement as it affects patients and their family/carers.

Reflective Activity 10.5

Re-read the case of Michael in Case Scenario 10.1 and consider the losses that might be experienced by his family and carers. Again, remember that losses can be physical, psychological, social and spiritual.
- What losses might be experienced by Michael's wife, Alicia?
- What losses might be experienced by his children, Aiden and Jennifer?
- Might the birth of the third child compensate Michael, Alicia or the children for the losses that they have experienced?

Common losses in similar circumstances could include loss of role, sense of purpose, income, activity, body image, physical relationship and status, all of which bring changes in relationships and roles and contribute to spiritual distress.

LOSS, GRIEF AND BEREAVEMENT IN PRACTICE

If a genuinely therapeutic, holistic environment is to be created, and if those experiencing the pain of loss are to find their spiritual destabilisation appropriately dealt with, such losses, and the feelings and expressions of grief which arise from them, have to be acknowledged, understood and responded to appropriately.

However, despite the expectation that healthcare professionals will support people who are struggling with loss, many will have had no formal education about the process of loss, grief and bereavement, or about appropriate responses which can be offered. Consequently, although it would not be appropriate to trap our thinking in one model or another so that a rigid and static view of the grief processes is created, or to seek to turn all healthcare professionals into mini bereavement counsellors, a review of grief theories as outlined above will help to form a deeper understanding of the grief process and provide a framework for clinical experiences and interventions.

In addition, a basic familiarisation with the issues will help healthcare professionals to become more aware of what they can offer in practice to help to communicate an understanding of the grief expressed, and to 'normalise' it in a helpful and supportive way. It will also allow an assessment to be made of any more worrying aspects of grief – what might loosely be called 'abnormal' or 'extreme' reactions – and to make appropriate referrals to more specialised resources. However, in the authors' experience, such abnormal reactions are very rare, and the spectrum of 'normality' is very wide indeed. Consequently, a predominant focus on the 'adverse' or 'extreme' reaction to loss over and against a 'normalising' approach can ultimately be unhelpful, as it can lead both to the 'pathologising' of grief, and to overlooking the more normal and typical reactions.

As seen in the reflections on Case Scenario 10.1, the loss of dignity, role, sexual expression of the depth of a relationship, routine, faith, hope, opportunities for the future, decision making, control, hope, and much more besides is important here. In this context, 'valuing the moment' in which reactions to losses are expressed in the context of a relational engagement with a healthcare professional is important.

Losses do not lend themselves to 'fixing' as is the case for much of what healthcare offers. What people who are experiencing loss desire most is for Bert or Jean not to be dead, for their disability to be taken away, for their terminal diagnosis to be a mistake, for their sorrow to be over, or for the use of their legs to return. In short, they want caring healthcare professionals to take their pain away. Recognition that this is not possible is, of course, where a continued engagement with the suffering of loss has to begin. However, bereaved people, and others expressing their losses in different ways, have often seen those to whom they reach out for understanding turn away in their uselessness, because they feel that they have nothing to offer if the ultimate is not available. Yet any healthcare professional who turns towards the broken and grieving person offers a powerful reassurance that all is not lost, and therefore helps to create an environment in which spiritual healing can take place.

Therefore 'valuing the moment', allowing the pain to be expressed and not feeling that it has to be either fixed or ignored, offers a greater depth of healing in the devastation of loss than many healthcare professionals might realise.

A good death

Research indicates that 'a good death', in the sense of a person being at peace and being 'whole' spiritually in their dying, provides a more solid platform for bereavement for those who are left.[13]

Case Scenarios 10.2 and 10.3 and Reflective Activity 10.6 will help us to explore our understanding of what a good death might or might not be, and its potential impact on spiritual distress and bereavement.

CASE SCENARIO 10.2

William is 78 years old and is in the end stages of lung cancer. He is an ex-miner, has defined himself as a Marxist and atheist, and exhibits an aggressive and uncompliant attitude to members of the healthcare team, particularly the female staff. In conversation with the social worker, he indicates that he is worried about his wife. When this is explored further, it becomes clear that William and his wife have not been able to talk openly about the terminal nature of his illness. The social worker facilitates a conversation between

(continued)

William and his wife in which more open and tender things are said by William than the social worker and William's wife expected. William dies a few days later, and appears to have had a more peaceful death than anyone expected. The social worker spends time with William's wife and family immediately after his death and during the following day as the paperwork and William's belongings are dealt with. William's wife and family express their gratitude that William's death was peaceful. His wife tells the social worker that she was pleased they had had a chance to talk together, and that 'William had a good end'.

CASE SCENARIO 10.3

Veronica has been largely unconscious since her family were informed that she was in the end stages of her illness. They had expected her to be around for longer, but the onset of unconsciousness, and the consequent indication of the closeness of the end, have taken everyone by surprise. Veronica's husband, Terry, had promised himself that they would talk together 'when the time was right', but now that there is no opportunity to do so, he is distraught that he has let her down and that he has no indications of what her wishes are with regard to a funeral. He has now been with her for almost three days. During that time he has had little sleep, and has only left her bedside to go home for a shower and a change of clothes. In her last hours, Veronica is experiencing what the doctor calls 'terminal agitation', and despite the reassurance of members of the healthcare team that 'she isn't suffering', her husband is deeply anxious that he can do nothing to help her. He pleads with the doctor to 'give her something' to ease her passing, and then immediately feels guilty about making this request. He tells anyone who will listen that 'you wouldn't let a dog die like this.' Veronica dies at 2.30 in the morning. Terry has been at her bedside all night, but had just gone to the toilet, and wasn't there when the end came. He has no knowledge, therefore, of what the end was like for his wife. The occupational therapist, who had been involved with Veronica and Bill for many months, spends time with Veronica's family the day after her death. However, she can have no constructive discussions of any meaningful kind with them because of Veronica's husband's distress about 'the hellishness of the end'.

Reflective Activity 10.6

Reflecting on Case Scenarios 10.2 and 10.3, and from your own experience of dealing with dying and death in your own clinical setting, list the factors that support or challenge a good death.

Supporting factors	*Challenging factors*

As experienced healthcare professionals, we might come to our own understanding of a good death based on our clinical experiences. However, as with all spiritual issues, only the individual can truly decide what is a good death.

Through a progressive approach to loss, grief and bereavement, we can use a basic understanding of theory alongside our experience to develop skills that will enable us to deal with the impact of loss and its contribution to spiritual distress, and to support the patients and their family and carers in our care.

CHAPLAIN OR SPIRITUAL CARE PROFESSIONAL

The expectation is that, as a spiritual care lead, the chaplain will either be formally involved with bereavement support networks or with grieving individuals, or will have to respond directly to referrals from members of the healthcare team who feel unable to respond adequately to bereavement needs which arise as part of their professional responsibilities. In this sense, the chaplain might be expected to act as a 'bereavement specialist' or, at the very least, to fulfil that role as and when demanding grief and bereavement situations arise.

Case Scenario 10.4 and Reflective Activity 10.7 will enable you to reflect on your practice from the perspective of your professional role as you consider how you might best facilitate good spiritual care in loss, grief and bereavement.

CASE SCENARIO 10.4

Wendy's husband, Victor, had died after a short and traumatic illness. Wendy was 58 years old, and she and her husband had been happily married for just over 33 years. Victor was a lawyer, and as the years had gone by he had built up not only a very successful business locally, but also a reputation in government circles relating to the field of European law. Wendy and Victor lived a comfortable although not ostentatious lifestyle, Wendy not having to work and seeing her role as a support to and companion for her husband. She travelled with him, she sat with him at official dinners, she hosted necessary cocktail parties, and she socialised at important functions. She organised his travel, and supported him on lecture tours and at the presentation of important papers and seminars. Wendy and Victor were inseparable. They had one daughter, Jennifer, who lived abroad and who, like her father, was a career lawyer. Victor had decided that he would retire at 60. After all, there would be no financial worries and, with more time together, he and Wendy could 'live off the fruits of their labours' and do all the things they had always wanted to do together. Their plans made them feel quite young again. Nine months before his sixtieth birthday, Victor saw his doctor about persistent headaches. Tests led to the diagnosis of a brain tumour. Within six months he was dead. Wendy was devastated. Although she was left comfortably well off, that counted for nothing compared with the loss of her whole reason for living. Death had destroyed the promise of what was to come. The partnership had been severed, and it was permanent. For Wendy, too, there was anger. It was a strange yet fundamentally understandable feeling, and in her case it was mostly directed at Victor. She didn't want to feel this way, but she simply couldn't help it. Victor had promised her so much, and now he had abandoned her and taken all the good stuff with him. She knew that it was irrational. But the heart that was broken was ferociously angry at the pain of loss, and the anger was directed at the one who had caused that pain.

Reflective Activity 10.7

Reflecting on Case Scenario 10.4, consider the following:
- What losses might Wendy be experiencing?
- What feelings might be associated with these losses?
- How would you describe the spiritual dimension of what Wendy is experiencing?

Utilising what you consider to be the grief theory most applicable to Wendy's situation:
- How might she expect to work towards a resolution of her grief?
- What might be offered to her to help her on this grief journey?
- What would you consider to be an appropriate outcome for Wendy?

Two things should be clear from this reflective activity. First, the feelings that Wendy had, including her negative feelings – particularly anger – towards her husband for leaving her 'and taking all the good stuff with him', are normal and appropriate in the devastation of bereavement. They are a threat to spiritual stability, in as much as they are a threat to meaning, purpose, fulfilment, hope and future plans. They create such feelings of dislocation from normality that bereaved people struggle to see how life can ever make any sense again, and how their 'destabilised' state will ever find equilibrium again. Finding a new sense of meaning after a loss is fundamental to the bereavement process. The beginning of that search for meaning is an acceptance of the reality of the pain and suffering that the loss brings.

Secondly, what Wendy was experiencing is classic in loss scenarios, as we have outlined earlier. If the loss of your car keys also brings with it the loss of being at the school on time, or missing the job interview, with the accompanying loss of face and self-worth, the same is true of bereavement. Wendy had lost her husband. So much is obvious. That is what bereavement means. However, she had also lost her role, her sense of purpose and her best friend, along with all the future plans which, given Victor's impending retirement, were if not almost reality in practice, certainly reality in Wendy's mind. Losses, therefore, are not single entities to be scrutinised as being one-dimensional and fitted into a prescribed theory or pattern. They are multi-faceted, and the losses which come with other losses are interwoven into a complex and tangled whole, which has to be accepted for what it is.

If the uniqueness of Wendy's confused pattern of interrelated losses has to be worked through, so the uniqueness of her place in that complex pattern has to be accepted, and her individual journey through bereavement understood and supported.

Losses are part of life. The reactions to them are not illnesses to be cured, but journeys to be followed. The 'why?' questions are not questions in the sense that they seek answers – they are cries of pain, and have to be responded to as such. The spiritual destabilising and dislocation that are experienced by those who struggle with loss can be understood, accepted and responded to appropriately, to the ultimate benefit of those who are grieving and, in addition, to the satisfaction of the healthcare professionals who are seeking to offer a holistic and spiritually aware and therapeutic environment.

In this context, the chaplain is often the first 'port of call' when bereavement issues arise. The upside of this is that the chaplain is perceived to be a 'safe pair of hands', and someone who understands the destabilising effects of loss, and the individuality of the journey of loss, grief and bereavement. The downside is that healthcare professionals, including chaplains, are not adequately equipped with a knowledge of grief theories and the uniqueness of the processes of grief and loss.

Two things follow, therefore, if the chaplain is to respond adequately to the complexities of bereavement issues. First, they must themselves be equipped for the task, for all the reasons outlined above. Secondly, if they are not, or if they do not have the capacity or resources to respond appropriately, they must be familiar with other support within and outside the healthcare setting, and be prepared to refer on when necessary.

FURTHER READING

➤ Investigate your local guidelines and protocols for bereavement services and find out what services for bereavement are available in your local area. Your local healthcare chaplain or social worker should be able to help.
➤ The Scottish Government's recommendations for bereavement support structures in health board areas: *Shaping Bereavement Care: consultation on a framework for action for bereavement care in NHS Scotland*. www.scotland.gov.uk/publications/2010/10/21155042/13 (accessed October 2010).
➤ National Institute for Clinical Excellence. *Improving Supportive and Palliative Care for Adults with Cancer. Manual*. London: National Institute for Clinical Excellence; 2004.
➤ The Scottish Government. *Living and Dying Well: a national action plan for palliative and end of life care in Scotland*. www.scotland.gov.uk/Publications/2008/10/01091608/11 (accessed January 2011).

REFERENCES

1 Freud S. Mourning and melancholia. In: Stratchey J (ed.) *The Standard Edition of the Works of Sigmund Freud*. London: Hogarth Press; 1957.
2 Lindemann E. Symptomatology and management of grief. *Pastoral Psychology* 1963; 14: 8–18.
3 Kübler-Ross E. *On Death and Dying*. London: Routledge; 1973.
4 Bowlby J. *Attachment and Loss. Volume 1. Attachment*. New York: Basic Books; 1969.
5 Bowlby J. *Loss: sadness and depression*. New York: Basic Books; 1970.
6 Bowlby J. *Attachment and Loss. Volume 2. Separation, anxiety and anger*. New York: Basic Books; 1973.
7 Parkes CM. *Bereavement: studies of grief in adult life*. London: Tavistock; 1972.

8 Worden JW. *Grief Counselling and Grief Therapy: a handbook for mental health practitioners*, 3rd edn. New York: Springer Publishing; 2002.

9 Klass D, Silverman P, Nickman S (eds) *Continuing Bonds: new understandings of grief.* Washington, DC: Taylor & Francis; 1996.

10 Gordon T. Recovering our lost saints: a current theory of loss and its Christian expression. *Scottish Journal of Healthcare Chaplaincy* 2004; **7**: 28–33.

11 Walter T. *On Bereavement; the culture of grief (facing death)*. Buckingham: Open University Press; 1999.

12 Stroebe M, Schut H. The dual process model of coping with bereavement: rationale and description. *Death Studies* 1999; **23**: 197–224.

13 Gordon T. *New Journeys Now Begin*. Glasgow: Wild Goose Publications; 2006.

CHAPTER 11

Nurturing our spiritual selves

INTRODUCTION

If self, our humanity, is the greatest resource that healthcare staff utilise in the provision of spiritual care, it follows that to maintain and develop best practice we need to nurture and take care of ourselves. More than that, there is a cost to delivering compassionate and person-centred spiritual care in complex situations of high expressed and felt emotion. It requires us to be vulnerable and open as human beings to the pain and distress of others. Being and waiting with others in times of transition, loss and uncertainty is draining emotionally, physically and spiritually. Being engaged in this way repeatedly without attention to these dimensions of our personhood can lead to increased levels of stress and burnout. This may reveal itself, for example, in a reduced sense of personal worth and effectiveness, exhaustion and increasingly negative perceptions about patients.[1] How do we as healthcare professionals and, importantly, as human beings process our experiences of supporting distressed service users and the emotions, issues and questions that are raised in us? Where is the balm in our lives to soothe and care for our souls? How may we learn and grow in an understanding of ourselves and our practice, as individuals and as teams working in relationship, from reflecting on experience? This chapter seeks to raise the key issue of well-being for healthcare staff, and to explore possibilities with regard to how we care for and develop our spiritual selves.

Reflective Activity 11.1 will remind you of some of the work done in connection with self-awareness in Chapter 1, and will help you to reflect on what contributes to your own particular well-being.

Self-awareness is a significant component of enabling a practitioner to provide sensitive person-centred spiritual care (as highlighted in Chapters 1 and 8). If as healthcare professionals our ability to deliver sensitive spiritual care involves our use of self as a therapeutic tool, then it follows that when we feel significantly disconnected or distracted, the care that we offer will be less effective. Therefore being aware of signs of stress within ourselves is as important as recognising our need to feel well and in what circumstances we tend to feel energised and really alive. Reflective Activity 11.2 is intended to help you to reflect on your level of awareness of how you exhibit signs of stress.

Reflective Activity 11.1

Make a list of moments in your life when you felt really alive. Next to those moments, note any associated factors or activities that contributed to such a feeling.

When I felt really alive	Associated factors or activities
For example, standing at the top of a mountain	Above the clouds, sheer beauty and quiet, long walk in, so a sense of achievement

- Do you ever feel fully alive at work? If so, when?
- When was the last time you felt really alive?
- What do you plan to do about this?

Reflective Activity 11.2

- What are the signs that you or others notice which indicate you are stressed?
- How does stress affect your behaviour and your ways of relating to others? For example, consider its effect on your emotions, mood, temperament, patience, etc.
- What short-term strategies do you use to help you to cope when you get stressed?

It is not just recognising when we are stressed that is important. It is also identifying the cause of our stress. This is what you are being encouraged to explore in Reflective Activity 11.3.

Reflective Activity 11.3

Make a list of what stresses you most at work, and then consider the impact of these stressors on you. For example, what feelings are associated with the stressors?

Stressors at work	Impact
For example, lack of communication between healthcare disciplines	Frustration, waste of time chasing up information

- Are there ways in which you might tackle any of the causes of stress?
- How might you minimise the impact on you of any stressors that you feel cannot be eradicated?

Undoubtedly, the culture in which healthcare staff work, the morale of the team or place of work, and the degree of willingness of colleagues to be open and supportive all affect our well-being. There will be some aspects of our workplace which we cannot change and others which we may be able to improve, often with the support of others. However, ultimately each of us has to take responsibility for our own well-being and make caring for ourselves, and not just for others, a priority. How we may do so is the focus of the rest of this chapter.

REFLECTING WITH OTHERS: A RANGE OF REFLECTIVE OPPORTUNITIES

There are a range of relationships or situations within which healthcare staff may actively reflect on their practice and experience, consciously or not, ranging from informal conversations to more disciplined and rigorous approaches. Chatting over the morning's events while having lunch or discussing the challenges of caring for a sick patient and his distressed relatives at a handover or multi-disciplinary meeting are significant ways in which practitioners process their experiences and deal with the impact of caring on themselves as human beings and healthcare professionals. With ever-increasing demands on staff, it is imperative that time is allowed for such exchanges to enable the sharing of stories, the safe discharge of feelings, and sometimes for humour to be found in a situation. A range of opportunities to reflect on spiritual care practice will be outlined here, starting with the more informal (but by no means less significant) ways.

Case Scenario 11.1 and Reflective Activity 11.4 will give you the opportunity to think about the possible benefits of reflecting with others, as well as the challenges of making reflective time and space work.

CASE SCENARIO 11.1

Enthused by their involvement in an interactive workshop exploring spiritual care in healthcare practice facilitated by a chaplain and an allied healthcare professional practice education facilitator, a small multi-disciplinary group of healthcare staff working in a local district general hospital began to meet informally to share their experiences of providing spiritual care. The group decided not to have a facilitator, but basic shared ground rules, such as confidentiality, were agreed upon. Participants brought their experiences and reflections to share informally with the rest of the group, who could respond as they felt appropriate. The group met once or twice a month over lunch, and interested parties came along as their other commitments allowed.

Reflective Activity 11.4

List the possible benefits (both professional and personal) to participants in the spiritual care reflective group outlined in Case Scenario 11.1.

Professional benefits	*Personal benefits*
For example, seeking advice from colleagues when dealing with a complex situation	Finding perspective if the practitioner feels that the wrong thing has been said or done

- What might be the challenges to individuals and the group as a whole to ensure that it continues and enables all those interested to benefit?

Undoubtedly, there are increasing difficulties for healthcare staff in finding time to reflect on practice, especially if the time is not protected and agreed upon with line managers. Informal and unstructured groups can potentially provide mutual support, and opportunities to externalise work-related issues and keep these in perspective. However, there is a danger of this being perceived as developing a clique, and without a facilitator there is a potential risk that groups can become dominated by strong personalities or particular topics, especially negative ones.

A similarly informal, yet intentional, way of reflecting on practice is the development of *critical conversation partnerships* or friendships. In this case, practitioners take responsibility for initiating regular meetings with a colleague whom they trust and whom they feel would not only affirm and listen to them, but also be honest enough to challenge or question practice or unhelpful rumination. Again, it would be important to discuss the basic ground rules of the relationship and clarify its purpose. A more formalised version of such relationships, which may be normative and expected within a healthcare context, depending on the culture of a ward, unit or healthcare discipline, is *mentoring* or *peer supervision*. Mentoring most commonly involves a relationship between a more experienced, reflective practitioner and a junior colleague within which practice and its effect on an individual's identity and well-being can be reflected upon. In the authors' experience, such arrangements are most effective when a healthcare professional has the opportunity to select a mentor, rather than such a relationship being prescribed. Peer supervision is a similar relationship, based on mutual trust and respect, in which growth and transformation may occur. It is intentionally created by two experienced practitioners who have a significant degree of self-awareness.

Supervision, either on a one-to-one basis or in a group, is a regular, planned, intentional and bounded space in which a practitioner skilled in supervision (the supervisor) meets with one or more other practitioners (the supervisees) to look together at the supervisees' practice.[2]

Pastoral supervision is becoming increasingly normative within healthcare chaplaincy, and may be of interest and benefit to other healthcare practitioners who wish their reflection on practice to include a theological dimension. As with other forms of supervision, pastoral supervision includes an element of account-ability and ensuring fitness to practise, as well as providing the opportunity for personal and professional growth and development.[3]

Supervision is not counselling, where there is a formalised relationship which seeks to help individuals to deal with particular areas of their life that they are finding challenging or destructive. However, supervisors may recommend that practitioners take particular issues to a counsellor. Nor is supervision spiritual direction, where individuals explore their relationship with God with a contemplative, wise 'other.' However, practitioners may well explore with a supervisor faith and belief issues that emerge from their practice.

Action learning sets offer another facilitated 'bounded space' in which healthcare staff can reflect on practice, and help complex situations or relationships to be understood more deeply and future practice informed (a fuller exploration of this reflective tool can be found in Chapter 12).

Reflective Activity 11.5 will help you to think about what makes someone an appropriate person to help you reflect on your practice. However, just as importantly, it will challenge you to explore what attributes and attitudes you require to get the most out of such a relationship.

Reflective Activity 11.5

- What makes a good critical friend or supervisor?
- What makes a good reflective practitioner?
- Whether you are religious or not, how do you respond to the essence of the following Sufi story retold by Mohammad Shabbir, the manager of a community development organisation which works with people living with mental health problems?[4]

When a novice came to a sheikh (teacher) and wanted to learn from him, the reply of the Sufi teacher was that in fact we are all students, and that the teacher is God. So there are no experts, only lives and journeys that need to be shared in order to find new meanings.

Part of what reflective practice involves, especially reflection on the provision of spiritual care, is being open to discovering new ways of understanding, interpret-ing and seeing for all involved, no matter how experienced, wise or well trained they may be. This in turn informs and potentially transforms the way of being and relating of all participants in their professional practice and personal lives. This is what has been described as a 'reflective cycle'. Such reflective practice can begin with what the writer and psychoanalyst, Patrick Casement, describes as 'internal supervision in process',[5] continues through learning from reflection on the engagement with the patient, and is worked out in the way that it informs future practice and personal development and growth.

Significant questions to consider when reflecting on spiritual care practice

No matter what kind of relationship or forum is utilised by a practitioner to reflect on spiritual care practice, there are a few key questions which are important to consider when exploring a particular experience or encounter with trusted others:

➤ What did that experience tell me about my ability to deliver sensitive spiritual care?

➤ What did it affirm about me, and what might I have to work on?

➤ How did the experience challenge, confront or make me explore my beliefs, values and understanding of the world, suffering, death and what may or may not be beyond?

➤ What did my practice tell me about myself and my identity (who I am, why I am as I am, and why I relate to others the way I do)?

➤ Whose needs were really being met in the situation we are considering (those of the patient, their carer, my colleagues, or my own)?

Reflection on practice does not just involve cognition. It potentially involves utilising all of our being and our senses. Spiritual care is delivered by embodied human beings, not just by professionals who only access their minds. Therefore rounded reflective practice involves, for example, expressing feelings as well as thoughts, being honest about touch, and verbalising our response to sights and smells, or possible feelings of sexual attraction or repulsion.

REFLECTIVE PRACTICE WRITING: EXAMPLES OF TOOLS THAT CAN BE UTILISED

> Reflective practice writing is a way of expressing and exploring our own and others' stories; crafting and shaping them to aid understanding and development.[6]

The first two examples of approaches to creative reflective practice include (but are not confined to) writing.

Critical incident analysis approach

Utilising particular tools to aid reflection, such as the critical incident analysis approach,[7] can be helpful for pre- and post-registration practitioners. Such reflective cycles can be used to aid reflection in small groups or as part of reflective writing exercises (e.g. by highlighting important aspects of caring for a dying patient in an intensive-care unit[8]). Such a methodology can help to enhance strategies for identifying and reflecting on practice strengths, weaknesses and obstacles (e.g. in developing leadership skills in nurses[9]).

Recreation of the imagined reality of an encounter

Kate Collier has developed a creative approach to workplace learning which helps practitioners to replay a specific situation in their mind, and then explore their inner imaginative playfulness with a colleague in order to develop a written case study and learn from the group discussion that follows.[10] Experimentally, she encouraged participants to visualise an encounter by re-creating it as if it was a play on stage, and engaging with the scenario like an audience at the theatre. In doing so, Collier's aim was to 'stimulate an aesthetic response from students and concentrate their focus and attention on the event so that it became more significant for them.'[10]

Verbatims

Emerging in the 1920s from the reflections of the American mental health chaplain, Anton Boisen, following his own experience of psychiatric illness, was the idea that pastors or chaplains in training should engage in the study of 'living human documents.'[11] Boisen was concerned that those seeking to care for others' spiritual needs should engage intentionally with patients' subjective lived experience, and not distance themselves from such experience by objectifying patients' stories by merely utilising theological language. Boisen was one of the father figures of the development of the Clinical Pastoral Education movement in the USA, which utilised the verbatim as a significant tool for facilitating reflective practice. Verbatims involve practitioners not only writing down word for word what they perceived to have been said during part of an encounter with a service user, but also noting their observations and reflections about what was seen, heard, felt and meant by both parties. Verbatims have been utilised as a significant resource to aid reflection on practice within supervision and reflective practice groups in clinical settings by various disciplines. Further details on writing verbatims can be found in *Helping the Helpers: Supervision in Pastoral Care*,[12] *Lifelong Learning: Theological Education and Supervision*[13] and *Pastoral Supervision: a Handbook.*[14]

Journaling

Learning journals are private places in which thoughts, feelings, insights, questions and new discoveries from practice can be laid out and reflected upon as they are written, or returned to at a later date. When recorded in a journal, snippets and nuggets of significant new understandings, mined from reflecting on the routine, the rewarding and the difficult, can be valuable resources for more public sharing and scrutiny in reflective groups:[15]

> By keeping a personal–professional journal you are both the learner and the one who teaches. You can chronicle events as they happen, have a dialogue with facts and interpretations, and learn from experience. A journal can be used for analysis and introspection. Reviewed over time it becomes a dialogue with

yourself. Patterns and relationships emerge. Distance makes new perspective possible: deeper levels of insight can form.

Reflective Activity 11.6

Select one of the reflective practice writing tools outlined above which is unfamiliar to you, and do some background reading about it. (Examples of background reading can be found in the Further Reading section at the end of this chapter).
- Select an experience, encounter or period of time from your spiritual care practice to reflect on utilising your chosen reflective methodology. Once you have performed your piece of reflective writing, share it with a trusted colleague, mentor or supervisor.
- To what extent did the tool enable you to reflect on your practice from a different angle or perspective?

Each of us will be naturally drawn to some particular reflective tools more than others, according to our own preferences and personalities. However, it is important as reflective practitioners to get into the habit of experimenting with a variety of approaches to performing reflective practice, to enable us to gain new perspectives and challenge what may be deeply held assumptions about the care that we offer.

RITUAL

In Chapter 8, the role of ritual in the provision of spiritual care to service users was explored. In addition, ritual has a potentially significant role for healthcare practitioners not only in the processing of loss and bereavement, but also in helping staff to find meaning and fulfilment in practice. The authors have always been slightly envious of nursing staff who are involved in the last act of care for a patient. While realising that this can be a potentially challenging experience, washing and spending time with a deceased person can allow stories and significant experiences to be shared, thus creating an opportunity to mark not just the life and death of the deceased, but the importance of your relationship with them for you, however fleeting it may have been.

Reflective Activity 11.7

- How do you acknowledge endings as part of your practice: for example, when patients die and their carers are no longer present on the ward or unit, especially those to whom you have become close or with whom you had an affinity?
- How do you acknowledge the significance and ending of such relationships?

One of the most significant, yet often unspoken, spiritual challenges for healthcare staff (including non-clinical staff) in our working lives, which affects our individual and shared communal well-being, is how we deal (or do not deal) with the accumulated losses and bereavements that we experience. It is the authors' experience that, on the whole, the traumatic, out-of-the-ordinary deaths and experiences of loss in healthcare settings are acknowledged and attempts at shared processing are usually made in wards, units and teams. This is done either through storytelling and conversation within formal or organised settings, or informally during or outside work. But what about the accumulated exposure to loss that goes un-named and unrecognised, and therefore remains unprocessed? What effect does constant exposure to loss have on each one of us, including, for example:

➤ the continuous ending of relationships with patients and their carers
➤ patients' loss of identity and sense of self
➤ patients' loss of physical body parts, mental faculties and control
➤ death, dying and bereavement?

Perhaps here, too, ritual can help. Case Scenario 11.2 gives a formal example of the role of ritual in processing loss. As you engage with it you might like to reflect on any personal or shared rituals that you perform or in which you have been involved that help you to deal with loss and bereavement.

CASE SCENARIO 11.2

John was a much loved member of the renal unit staff in the teaching hospital in which he worked. He had worked there for over 15 years, first as a specialist registrar and then as consultant nephrologist. Sadly, he died suddenly at the age of 47 from a heart attack. The whole unit was shocked and badly shaken by his death. Three weeks after John's funeral, over a cup of coffee in the staffroom, one of John's colleagues asked the hospital chaplain if she would help the unit to celebrate John's life with a short memorial service, as well as help them to deal with the sense of unreality of what had happened. The feeling in the unit was that the funeral had not really done John's colourful and lively personality justice, as well as the significance of his contribution to the life and well-being of the unit. John was divorced and lived alone, and had no children. His funeral had been planned by his brother, to whom he had not been close, and was conducted by a local minister who hadn't known John at all. The John whose life and death had been marked at the crematorium was not the John that his colleagues knew.

The chaplain was more than happy to work with different members of staff to enable them to create a fitting ritual to enact their relationship with John and his significance to them, his patients and their carers, and the unit as a whole. During the service the feeling of sadness and loss, although broken at times by much shared laughter, prompted by staff reminiscences of John, was palpable. In response to this and her own inner dialogue, the chaplain found herself acknowledging that what was happening was not just a pausing from the routine and the busyness of days and weeks in the renal unit to remember John. In doing so, individually and together, she and her colleagues were recognising and expressing feelings associated with countless accumulated, buried, unprocessed and unnamed losses.

(continued)

> *In the week following the memorial service, a small contingent of nursing staff from the unit came into the chaplain's office and asked if she might help them to hold an annual service during which staff could acknowledge and have some space to help process the losses that they and their colleagues experienced as part of their working lives.*

Ritual enables the public recognition of loss and endings. Such shared marking of endings and losses not only enables feelings to be discharged, but also allows the significance of relationships and the professional and personal meaning that is found in them to be acknowledged.

PLAY

It is not just as children that we express ourselves through play. Much meaning and purpose can be found in life, as well as the expression of feelings and the discovery of insights, through play. Play can be physical, musical, lyrical, creative or imaginative, but whatever our particular choice of activity, it should always be fun. Each of us likes to play in different ways, and how we play changes with age, circumstances and mood. Play is often part of what enlivens human relationships and our engagement with the world around us, within us and beyond us. It is essential for our spiritual well-being, both in order to feed our souls and to enable us to continue to care for others in an ongoing way.

Reflective Activity 11.8 is designed to make you consider how you express the playful part of your nature – a significant yet often ignored aspect of our humanity.

Reflective Activity 11.8

- How do you play?
- Do you dance, make or listen to music, garden, play sport, write, draw or paint?
- When was the last time you played?
- How playful are the significant relationships in your life?
- When was the last time you really laughed (on your own, at yourself or with others)?

SILENCE

In our modern urban lifestyles, silence can be an unusual and even counter-cultural experience. As a result, many of us can feel uncomfortable with silence in our life. Even if we are alone in our home, in our car or out walking, we often have the radio, television or our iPod for company.

If we are not comfortable with quiet, how can we make space for silence in our professional caring relationships? How can we be silent enough to listen, silent when there is no answer or nothing to say, and silent enough to enable other people to express themselves as they need to in the present moment? If we are comfortable with being quiet, this will often put others at ease, too:[16]

> However, it is not so much the absence of noise that enables connection – especially with the other – but stillness. Stillness is a state of attentiveness: 'It involves an awareness of one's being, not one's doing. That is why it is still. Silence is defined from outside, stillness from within.

Silence and stillness are not just important to practise if we wish to enhance our ability to be with and relate sensitively to service users in times of distress and uncertainty. They are also a significant means by which we can enhance how we relate intra-personally, inter-personally and trans-personally in every part of our lives. Some individuals and traditions will meditate, pray or use relaxation techniques that enhance the ability to be silent and inwardly still.

The following simple reflective activity is designed to help you to be quiet and still.

Reflective Activity 11.9

- Sit upright in a comfortable chair in a quiet room with your feet squarely on the ground and your hands relaxed and open on your lap.
- Place a candle, flowers, a plant, a stone, a photograph, a postcard or another suitable object on a table or on the floor in front of you, so that you can focus on it. If the weather is good you can try the same exercise on a park bench or in the garden.
- Relax and let the chair take your weight. Then breathe gently in through your nose and out through your mouth. It may help to concentrate on your breathing. If your thoughts drift, bring them back gently to focus on the object in front of you.
- Try this for 5 minutes at first, then perhaps for 10 or 15 minutes as you get more comfortable with being still.

Being still is not just about keeping our body in one position. It involves a centring and stillness within us which enable receptivity to the stories and feelings of others.

RHYTHM TO LIFE

Reflective Activity 11.10 is designed to help you to think about the balance in your life and how often you have the energy, time or space to be attentive to the present moment. In other words, how often do you really connect with the world around you and within you as part of nurturing your own spirituality?

Reflective Activity 11.10

Take time to slowly read through William Henry Davies' poem *Leisure* two or three times.[17] Pay attention to the thoughts, feelings and questions that arise within you as you do so. Note them down. What are these jottings saying to you about the rhythm of, or balance in, your life?

What is this life if, full of care,
We have no time to stand and stare.

No time to stand beneath the boughs
And stare as long as sheep or cows.

No time to see, when woods we pass,
Where squirrels hide their nuts in grass.

No time to see, in broad daylight,
Streams full of stars, like skies at night.

No time to turn at Beauty's glance,
And watch her feet, how they can dance.

No time to wait till her mouth can
Enrich that smile her eyes began.

A poor life this if, full of care,
We have no time to stand and stare.

CHAPLAIN OR SPIRITUAL CARE PROFESSIONAL

Healthcare chaplains, as discussed in Chapter 12, have a key role in supporting staff who are working in different healthcare contexts. Well-being in the workplace can only be meaningfully promoted by a chaplain who not only talks 'a good game' but actually embodies what he or she encourages others to embrace. In the authors' personal experience, it is far easier for chaplains to live out the maxim 'Do as I say, not as I do!' The final reflective activity in this chapter requires us as chaplains to closely review how we approach our ongoing spiritual and human development, to ask ourselves to what extent we process our experience of handling loss and bereavement, and whether we facilitate or deaden well-being in others and in our place of work by what we embody.

Reflective Activity 11.11

Take time to re-read this chapter again thoughtfully, and in doing so consider in particular the following questions:
• What makes you feel fully alive? How can you give yourself more opportunities to feel this way?
• How often do you get stressed?
  – Is there a pattern to this?

(continued)

- What can you do to remedy this if stress is significantly impinging on your quality of life and work?
- To what extent do the reflective/supervisory mechanisms that you have in place meet your real needs? Is there room and permission for wrestling, questioning, laughing and, at times, raging?
  - Do you need to change your method or pattern of reflecting or who you reflect with?
  - Can you be more creative and bold in your reflective practice? If so, how?
- How have your beliefs, values and self-understanding changed in the last 5 years?
  - How do you nurture your faith and beliefs?
- Honestly, how often do you really play, and how?
- When was the last time you were still and silent for 15 minutes?
- What aspects of your spiritual life need some gentle attention? Take time to make an action plan that is realistic and for future review.

As chaplains, like many in the caring professions, we can be more gentle with others than we are with ourselves. It is significant that others in healthcare may feel that they have permission to prioritise care for themselves if we, too, are able to do that for ourselves.

FURTHER READING

This reading will assist you with your chosen topic in Reflective Activity 11.6, and will also help you to explore different methods of reflection.

Critical incident analysis
➤ Fornasier D. Teaching ethical leadership through the use of critical incident analysis. *Creative Nursing* 2008; **14**: 116–21.
➤ Gould B, Masters H. Learning to make sense: the use of critical incident analysis in facilitated reflective groups of mental health students. *Learning in Health and Social Care* 2004; **3**: 53–63.
➤ Mulligan A. Should dying patients be monitored? A reflective analysis of a critical incident. *Nursing in Critical Care* 2005; **10**: 122–6.

Recreation of imagined reality encounter
➤ Collier K. Re-imagining reflection: creating a theatrical space for the imagination in productive reflection. In: Bradbury H, Frost N, Kilminster S, Zukas M (eds) *Beyond Reflective Practice: new approaches to professional lifelong learning.* London: Routledge; 2010. pp. 145–54.

Verbatims
➤ Leach J. Pastoral theology as attention. *Contact* 2007; **153**: 19–32.
➤ Leach J, Paterson M. *Pastoral Supervision: a handbook.* London: SCM Press; 2010.
➤ Ward F. *Lifelong Learning: theological education and supervision.* London: SCM Press; 2005.

Journaling
➤ Bolton G. *Reflective Practice: writing and professional development,* 2nd edn. London: Sage Publications Ltd; 2005.

➤ Lauterbach S, Hentz P. Journaling to learn: a strategy in nursing education for developing the nurse as person and person as nurse. *International Journal of Human Caring* 2005; **9**: 29–35.

➤ Van Horn R, Freed S. Journaling and dialogue pairs to promote reflection in clinical nursing education. *Nursing Education Perspectives* 2008; **29**: 220–25.

For more general reading on the topic we would recommend the following:

➤ Graham E, Walton H, Ward F. *Theological Reflection: methods.* London: SCM Press; 2005.

➤ Hawkins P, Shohet R. *Supervision in the Helping Professions,* 3rd edn. Buckingham: Open University Press; 2007.

➤ Stairs J. *Listening for the Soul: pastoral care and spiritual direction.* Minneapolis, MN: Fortress Press; 2000.

REFERENCES

1 Firth-Cozens J, Cornwell J. *The Point of Care: enabling compassionate care in acute hospital settings.* London: The King's Fund; 2009.

2 Association of Pastoral Supervisors and Educators (APSE). www.pastoralsupervision. org.uk (accessed February 2011).

3 Leach J, Paterson M. *Pastoral Supervision: a handbook.* London: SCM Press; 2010.

4 Shabbir M. Values and supervision. *Contact* 2006; **151**: 26.

5 Casement P. *On Learning from the Patient.* London: Routledge; 1985.

6 Bolton G. *Reflective Practice: writing and professional development,* 2nd edn. London: Sage Publications Ltd; 2005. p. 23.

7 Gould B, Masters H. Learning to make sense: the use of critical incident analysis in facilitated reflective groups of mental health students. *Learning in Health and Social Care* 2004; **3**: 53–63.

8 Mulligan A. Should dying patients be monitored? A reflective analysis of a critical incident. *Nursing in Critical Care* 2005; **10**: 122–6.

9 Fornasier D. Teaching ethical leadership through the use of critical incident analysis. *Creative Nursing* 2008; **14**: 116–21.

10 Collier K. Re-imagining reflection: creating a theatrical space for the imagination in productive reflection. In: Bradbury H, Frost N, Kilminster S, Zukas M (eds) *Beyond Reflective Practice: new approaches to professional lifelong learning.* London: Routledge; 2010. p. 150.

11 Gerkin C. *The Living Human Document: re-visioning pastoral counselling in a hermeneutical mode.* Nashville, TN: Abingdon Press; 1984.

12 Foskett J, Lyall D. *Helping the Helpers: supervision in pastoral care.* London: SPCK; 1988.

13 Ward F. *Lifelong Learning: theological education and supervision.* London: SCM Press; 2005.

14 Leach J, Paterson M. *Pastoral Supervision: a handbook,* op. cit.

15 Bolton G. *Reflective Practice: writing and professional development,* op. cit., p. 166.

16 Smith H, Smith M. *Helping Others: being around, being there, being wise.* London: Jessica Kingsley Publishers; 2008. p. 103.

17 BBC Books. *The Nation's Favourite Poems.* London: BBC Books; 1996. p. 32.

CHAPTER 12

The institution and staff support

INTRODUCTION

As has been explored in detail in Chapter 1, we are all spiritual beings, and consequently we have to be aware of our own spirituality in our engagement with those in our care who have spiritual needs. However, spiritual issues are often seen to be 'separate' and sometimes 'private' aspects of our lives, and therefore not integrated into our daily living and workplace environment. We set our spirituality in a separate compartment, which often means that we don't speak about it in the work setting. The Foundation for Workplace Spirituality suggests that although in the workplace we talk of 'team spirit' and 'the spirit of the company', we rarely link these terms to the underlying essence of spirituality, nor do we encourage spiritual practices in the workplace.[1] It asserts that 'Honouring our spiritual nature in the workplace is not only good for our souls (and psyche), but also good for the workplace, too.'

In addition, the team setting of the healthcare environment as outlined in Chapter 4 lends itself to the identification of and need to respond to issues of a spiritual nature. Consequently, the setting in which many healthcare professionals operate creates an environment in which there is a challenge to the compartmentalisation of our own spiritual issues, particularly where they relate to our well-being, and therefore potentially threaten the effective delivery of the services that we are charged with providing.

THE OPERATIONAL CONTEXT

It is clear that there have to be agreed standards of professional practice, both for the safety and well-being of patients and carers, and to allow for the auditing of the efficacy of service delivery. However, there will have to be standards which relate to the institution itself, including 'workplace spirituality', and the integral and supportive role that the chaplain has with regard to the rest of the healthcare team.

All staff who are working at any level with spiritual distress and seeking to offer spiritual care should have access to personal and professional support. The nature and delivery of spiritual care require the kind of self-awareness that was explored in Chapter 1 and was further examined in relation to the processing of a personal spiritual journey in Chapter 11. Such issues of self-awareness and spiritual growth will raise questions for healthcare professionals relating to clinical practice, personal worth, issues of life stance and coping strategies. Although there are a variety of services which staff may access outside work, there are aspects of support which remain integral to the work setting and to the way that the healthcare team operates.

Clearly, colleagues should and do support each other. In a context where openness is encouraged, there will be informal opportunities for support (debriefing, an encouraging word, etc.). However, more formalised support structures are also important. One such activity is 'action learning sets', which provide individual and organisational development. Members of staff work in small groups tackling important organisational issues or problems. In these groups they are able to learn from their attempts to change things. Action learning brings people together to exchange, support and challenge each other in seeking to act and learn.[2] Where such opportunities for supportive exploration exist, the spirituality of the individual is enhanced (e.g. in terms of meaning, self-worth, confidence and coping strategies). As a result, the individual feels supported, and the well-being of the institution is further strengthened. Much is being done to ensure that the healthcare team operates in a healthy and effective context if healthcare staff:

➤ are enabled to apply the principles of evidence-based practice in healthcare settings
➤ are focused on identifying, appraising and incorporating the results of medical and social research into the day-to-day practice and commissioning decisions
➤ are encouraged to learn how to implement the findings of research in practice to improve healthcare and the well-being of the organisation
➤ can identify gaps in evidence where further research is needed to inform commissioning decisions and the support structures required.[3]

TEAM SUPPORT

The healthcare team should therefore have regular opportunities for meeting together to explore all aspects of teamworking, both clinical and relational, to further develop good working practices and create and enhance a more satisfying working environment, ultimately and most importantly to the overall benefit of the holistic care that is offered to patients and their carers. Effective use of such opportunities builds trust, offers support, and allows individuals within the team to feel that they are both understood and cared for. However, notwithstanding the necessity for the team to meet together for support, the team context will also be such that stresses within the team can be acknowledged in their immediacy, faced up to and dealt with appropriately.

Case Scenario 12.1 and Reflective Activity 12.1 will guide you in thinking through aspects of spiritual support for members of the healthcare team.

CASE SCENARIO 12.1

The team members are assembled at a clinical meeting. There is discussion of the distressing case of a patient who has just received news that her son has been killed in a motor-cycle accident. Given the team's awareness of the emotional issues for the patient, the practical aspects of what needs might require to be processed and referred on, and the overall effect of this on the well-being of the patient and her journey to wholeness, appropriate decisions are made and necessary actions agreed, designated and recorded. There is a palpable sense of 'heaviness' among the team as they break up after the meeting. On returning to the ward, one of the nurses is found in tears in the duty room.

Reflective Activity 12.1

From your own experience and reflecting on Case Scenario 12.1, how would you respond to the following questions:
- What might your initial reaction be to finding the nurse in tears?
- What might be the cause of the nurse's distress?
- How might the nurse be supported?
- What about other members of the team who have not been found in tears in the duty room? What might their needs be, and how might they be supported?

Healthcare professionals are not machines, or human beings who encase themselves in a suit of armour so that they are always protected from the human feelings that are fundamental to the healthcare setting and good clinical practice. We need to remember that we are individuals with our own life experiences and needs as well as being healthcare professionals. It is not uncommon for current or past experiences from our personal life to bring out emotions that catch us by surprise and 'slip under our defences' or challenge our professional composure. There are some who may give the impression that they are immune from such personal influences, and that 'feelings' or human reactions are inappropriate and unprofessional. However, for most sensitive healthcare practitioners, feelings will continue to matter and will have to be processed, while they still remain professional and fully engaged with their duties and responsibilities.

BEING HONEST ABOUT FEELINGS AND EMOTIONS

It is inevitable that deep feelings and high-running emotions will at times be part of the healthcare context. Consequently, there are a number of things which should be clearly understood in the creation of a context of the mutuality of support. The first of these is seeing the expression of feelings as an indication of our humanity, and not construing such honesty and self-awareness as weakness or failure. Vulnerability is part of what we are and who we are.

Case Scenario 12.2 and Reflective Activity 12.2 will help you to think through personal and professional feelings and support.

CASE SCENARIO 12.2

This is a reflective account written by a charge nurse of an incident experienced in a care-of-the-elderly ward.

Marion was 85 years old, and was slowing dying from dementia-related issues. Her husband, Norman, and their daughter, Anne, were constant companions at her bedside. Circumstances meant that Marion had been on the unit for 4 months, and she had become a favourite of all the team. Many people were appropriately involved with her physical, emotional, psychological and spiritual care. People were touched by her humour, tenderness, compliance and ready smile, and by the clear expressions of the depth of the relationships between Marion, Norman and Anne. The team were, as usual, supportive of one another. There were days when some coped better than others, and there were other days when everyone felt down. It had been agreed by the team that Marion was dying, and she had been placed on the Liverpool Care Pathway.[4] When I came into the unit on the Monday morning after a weekend off, I was met at the back door by one of the healthcare assistants, who was sheltering in the doorway, having an 'illegal' cigarette. She was crying. When she saw me she didn't bother trying to explain the smoke, nor did she have to tell me what had happened, but she just fell into my arms and sobbed on my shoulder.

After a while, I left her to finish her cigarette and went up to the unit. Norman and Anne were in the room with Marion, the nurses having completed their 'final offices', and there were a lot of tears when I arrived. After a long time, Norman and Anne decided that it would be best to start thinking about moving on, and they began to take down the photographs, cards and other items from the walls of the room, and removed the personal knick-knacks from the locker. In the midst of all of this, the door opened and into the room came a distressed woman, who turned out to be Marion's younger sister, who had travelled from France to be with her sister before she died. On experiencing her distress, I also started to cry. I decided to slip out of the room to compose myself, and hoped that I could find a quiet corner where no one would notice me. But as soon as I stepped into the corridor, I bumped into the same healthcare assistant whom I had been comforting earlier. When she saw my distress, she put her arms around me and said 'So now it's your turn', and held me until my tears subsided. Then we smiled at each other and went our different ways.

Reflective Activity 12.2

Reflecting on your own experiences of expressions of emotion in your healthcare setting, and on the case outlined in Case Scenario 12.2, consider the following:
- How do you feel about and internally respond to this case scenario?
- How does this relate to your experience of dealing with distressing situations?
- How might the events surrounding Marion's illness and death be further explored for the benefit of the team?

Emotions and feelings are part of who we are as individuals, and often their expression is more about sincerity and honesty than about a break in a professional façade. Mutuality in the team context is important. Feelings can be talked about, worked through and understood, and when the environment encourages an honest sharing, this can be a very effective and supportive tool. Therefore the expression of feelings, far from exhibiting weakness, can actually provide opportunities for personal and corporate growth and support. However, in the context of this mutual support, such moments of honest sharing should be kept in confidence.

It would be hoped, for example, that the charge nurse in Reflective Activity 12.1 would be able to be honest about the source of her feelings of distress without this being held against her or her being regarded as someone who 'wasn't coping' or who had 'something wrong with her.' Similarly, it would be hoped that the emotion shared between a charge nurse and a healthcare assistant, and the appropriateness of their support for one another in their distress, would strengthen their understanding of one another and the mutuality of their professional engagement within the team.

Reflective Activity 12.3

Go back to Case Scenario 12.2 and Reflective Activity 12.2 and consider the positive and negative outcomes from the following questions:
- If confidentiality was breached or the feelings of either party were talked about in a negative way, what might be the threat to the working relationship between the charge nurse and the healthcare assistant, and ultimately the working relationships among the whole team?
- How might the individuals involved, and the team itself, build on the circumstances of this event?

Our level of performance can be threatened when the spirituality of the institution is unhealthy. Our level of service delivery, and our ability to cope with the stresses of our working context, depend on our ability to continue to function both in a professional manner appropriate to our roles and responsibilities, and in a personal framework that remains human and healthy. If the context of service delivery is compromised, the delivery of care will itself be challenged. On the other hand, the creation of a climate where feelings are recognised as important, and the enhancing of an environment in which emotions can be explored and worked through, continue to provide a working context in which honesty, support and personal well-being are important norms.

THE CHAPLAIN OR SPIRITUAL CARE PROFESSIONAL

While staff support and institutional practice are an important component of spiritual care for all healthcare professionals, they are designated a core area for healthcare chaplaincy in the *Spiritual and Religious Care Capabilities and Competences for Healthcare Chaplains*.[5,6] The specific place of chaplaincy in these areas is outlined clearly in the capability statements:

> ➤ **Staff support.** The chaplain builds working relationships with mem-
> bers of staff and volunteers and responds to requests for personal and
> professional support.
> ➤ **Chaplain to the hospital or unit.** The chaplain is aware of his or her role
> in the hospital or unit's major incident plan and responds to staff issues and
> events that need a communal recognition and action.[7]

What does this mean in practice? There will be times when staff turn to a designated member of the team for specific individual or team-related support. Those who provide such support should have that role outlined in their job description and professional competences. They should have well demarcated boundaries to their staff support role, and such support should not be confused with or seen as a substitute for good line management and appropriate appraisal processes, and should remain separate from any disciplinary issues.

The UK Board of Healthcare Chaplaincy acknowledges in its *Spiritual and Religious Care Capabilities and Competences for Healthcare Chaplains* that, in terms of 'institutional practice', the chaplain has a vital staff support role.[8] It states unequivocally that, as far as staff support is concerned, 'The chaplain builds working relationships with members of staff and volunteers and responds to requests for personal and professional support.' This support is underpinned by a working knowledge of the spiritual needs of healthcare professionals, an awareness of workplace stress and personal stress, and familiarity with the literature on provision of staff support, spiritual and religious care, or counselling skills. The support itself is demonstrated by a chaplain:

➤ building working relationships with staff, volunteers and groups
➤ respecting confidence in responding to requests for personal support from
members of staff and volunteers
➤ responding to requests for professional support from members of staff and
volunteers (e.g. by providing advice on and understanding of spiritual and
religious care, ethical issues or care issues)

➤ recognising his or her own personal skills and limitations in providing personal and professional support
➤ identifying other sources of internal or external staff support and, with the staff member's permission, facilitating referral.

Staff support can be in the hands of several key people (e.g. team leaders or ward managers), with the chaplain exercising responsibilities alongside and not instead of such roles. However, wherever the support role is located, it is underpinned by three factors:
➤ It is to be understood and responded to in a context of mutuality (i.e. with members of the team supporting one another).
➤ People in positions of responsibility also need support from the team.
➤ There will inevitably be times when it falls to one person to exercise a key role in the support of an individual, the whole team or the institution itself.

In addition, services users within the context of their care cannot be immune to aspects of organisational stress related to major events which affect the institution and the whole team, or as a result of an accumulation of aspects of a series of difficult situations which have to be responded to.

As was indicated earlier, where the chaplain is integrated into the multidisciplinary team and has a close working relationship with the other team members, it is right and proper that he or she should be designated as holding a staff support role. This is often separate from a management structure, for example, where the chaplain is the staff support person and a ward manager has appropriate line-management responsibility for a member or members of staff. As in Reflective Activity 12.1, when there are circumstances where the staff support role, in the immediacy of a stressful situation or as integral to someone's job description, is held by a member of the team who also carries management responsibilities, the two roles should be clearly delineated. The person seeking support should understand what 'hat' the supportive staff person is wearing at any given time.

Similarly, and perhaps more importantly, staff support and engagement with disciplinary processes should be distinct from each other.

Case Scenario 12.3 and Reflective Activity 12.4 will encourage you to explore these issues.

CASE SCENARIO 12.3

Tomasz is a recent immigrant with his wife from Poland, and works as a domestic in a busy Accident and Emergency department. Like most of his colleagues, he knows the chaplain well, as there is often a need for the chaplain to come to A&E for emergencies and to support distressed patients and family members. Over a two-year period Tomasz has grown to like and respect the chaplain, and has recently confided in her about his concerns

(continued)

for his wife, who has had a series of miscarriages. She has recently been in the neonatal unit, and not only has the chaplain visited her there, but she has also been supportive of Tomasz through stressful times. One day when Lucy, the chaplain, is in the department, Tomasz takes her aside and tells her that the next day he is to go for a meeting with his line manager and someone from Human Resources, to discuss a disciplinary issue concerning lateness and inadequate working. He asks Lucy if she will accompany him to the meeting, to assist with language issues and to offer him support, as he has no one else to turn to.

Reflective Activity 12.4

Reflecting on the case of Tomasz in Case Scenario 12.3 and your own professional role, consider your response to the following questions:
* What is the chaplain's role in relation to Tomasz?
* What might she decide to do?
* What might be the criteria on which she bases her decision?

It is not always easy for the chaplain to discern his or her distinct role. Such discernment is sometimes worked out in the immediacy of a situation or encounter, with no time or space to ponder, reflect or work out a careful strategy. There should be two guiding principles, namely what is best for Tomasz, and what appropriately keeps the relationship with him intact. Lucy's response will therefore be informed by her desire to:

➤ clarify boundaries with Tomasz
➤ ascertain which of his needs she can handle, and which might be best 'divided off' and referred to someone else
➤ help Tomasz to understand what his own roles and responsibilities are
➤ be aware of the ongoing needs of Tomasz and his wife
➤ 'keep the door open' to further pastoral care.

The chaplain cannot and should not be 'all things to all people', even though there may be times when that is an expectation which is expressed to the chaplain by individuals or the team. Consequently, Lucy needs to be aware of her personal and professional limitations, the team context, the working environment and necessary protocols, and her own well-being, in order to discern in the immediacy of this pastoral encounter what might be appropriate.

Reflective Activity 12.5

From your own experience, consider the following questions:
* What might be other circumstances in which a team member approaches the chaplain for support?
* What might be the chaplain's expected response?

The context in which the chaplain operates should always inform the response to the needs of the team and individuals within it. The chaplain is not a 'rescuer' or spiritual 'superhero', but an important level of support for and *within* the team setting. In addition, the level of support, and the appropriate expressions of that support, should not be static or inflexible, but should be adaptable to the needs of the situation and/or of the individual as these are presented or expressed.

FURTHER READING

For all healthcare professionals
➤ Foundation for Workplace Spirituality. www.workplacespirituality.org.uk/welcome (accessed January 2011).
➤ NHS Confederation. www.nhsconfed.org (accessed January 2011).
➤ Pedlar M. *Action Learning for Managers*. Aldershot: Gower Publishing Company; 2008.

For healthcare chaplains
➤ UK Board of Healthcare Chaplaincy. *Spiritual and Religious Capabilities and Competences for Healthcare Chaplains*. www.ukbhc.org.uk/publications/competencies (accessed February 2011).
Familiarise yourself with the 'Staff support' section on page 21 of this document, and complete a self-assessment of your competence.

REFERENCES

1 Foundation for Workplace Spirituality. www.workplacespirituality.org.uk/welcome (accessed January 2011).
2 Pedlar M. *Action Learning for Managers*. Aldershot: Gower Publishing Company; 2008.
3 NHS Confederation. www.nhsconfed.org (accessed January 2011).
4 Marie Curie Palliative Care Institute. *The Liverpool Care Pathway for the Dying Patient (LCP)*. Liverpool: Marie Curie Palliative Care Institute; 2009.
5 NHS Education for Scotland. *Spiritual and Religious Care Capabilities and Competences for Healthcare Chaplains*. Edinburgh: NHS Education for Scotland; 2008.
6 UK Board of Healthcare Chaplaincy. *Spiritual and Religious Care Capabilities and Competences for Healthcare Chaplains*. Cambridge: UK Board of Healthcare Chaplaincy; 2009.
7 UK Board of Healthcare Chaplaincy. *Spiritual and Religious Care Capabilities and Competences for Healthcare Chaplains*, op. cit.
8 UK Board of Healthcare Chaplaincy. *Spiritual and Religious Care Capabilities and Competences for Healthcare Chaplains*, op. cit., p. 22.

CHAPTER 13

Chaplain to the institution

INTRODUCTION

In Chapter 4 we concluded that no chaplain or spiritual care lead can operate without an awareness of the rest of the healthcare team, the corollary being that no chaplain can disregard the unit or institutional context in which the healthcare team is set. In addition, the chaplain, operating at the top level of competency in spiritual matters, will naturally be identified as the team member to whom others will look for support for their own spiritual issues.

If staff are to be encouraged to express their spirituality through the holistic model of health in caring for patients, the organisation itself must reflect those same core spiritual attitudes and values towards its staff.[1] Thus those responsible for the healthcare context should demonstrate their commitment to a 'spirituality of the organisation'. Such care is not only for patients. It includes staff and volunteers as well. As a result, there is an important role for the chaplain as 'chaplain to the institution' as a whole, as well as a support for individuals within it, as has been outlined in Chapter 12.

ORGANISATIONAL SPIRITUALITY

Organisational spirituality can be defined as 'enabling each employee to be able to realise their highest human potential, by embodying spiritual values and attitudes within the workplace, such as meaning, love, compassion, acceptance, forgiveness, value, and integrity.'[2] There are a number of discernible benefits of a more positive workplace spirituality, where staff are valued and find meaning in their daily work. *Spiritual Care Matters* suggests that there can be a release of human potential, such that staff bring their 'whole person' to work, using their innate strengths of creativity and empathy in their working relationships.[3] There can be an enhancement of a culture of 'service' to other staff and the organisation, rather than competition or undermining. In addition, staff can find 'meaning' in the workplace situation, which leads to improved personal job satisfaction, and lower rates of workplace stress and absenteeism. There can also be an improved performance of the organisation, with lower levels of staff turnover and better recruitment.

The *Spiritual Care Matters* guidance goes on to indicate that, as a result, there should be discernible signs of a flourishing organisational spirituality, which might include:

➤ policies and procedures of the organisation promoting a culture of personal growth, self-knowledge, and the maintenance of integrity

➤ staff enabled to create and achieve influence in their daily work

➤ the organisation having shared values which generate not only supportive relationships between staff, but also a sense of belonging and meaning

➤ leaders who, by demonstrating courage, creativity, sensitivity and empathy, have the ability to inspire other staff to reach their potential

➤ the presence of an active and effective staff support system.

> It is now widely accepted that those organisations which have a 'spiritually-friendly' culture show universally lower than average rates of absenteeism, workplace stress and staff turnover. 'Spiritual cultures' also provide opportunities for transcendence and interconnectedness through the work process which, within a moral framework, results in increased and better output. Thus workplace spirituality is not only good for the 'soul', but is also good for the workplace itself.[4]

INSTITUTIONAL STRESS

Throughout healthcare there are times of stress and difficulty, either related to major events which affect the institution and the whole team, or as a result of an accumulation of responses to a series of difficult situations, which have to be responded to. It is therefore important that there are structures in place to recognise times and events that cause institutional stress, to have standards and procedures in place to deal with them, and to be aware of who would be expected to take the lead in such situations.

Of course in any large institution there will be a plan in place which will outline the appropriate response to a major incident, and within such a plan there will be roles designated that will enshrine actions to be taken on behalf of the whole institution. In addition, there are national guidelines which offer clear pathways for supporting those who have experienced trauma, as victims and carers, as well as institutions as a whole. For example, the *NHS Emergency Planning Guidance* published by the Department of Health[5] offers national strategic guidance on planning for the psychological and mental health of people affected by major incidents and disasters.

Many of the causes of institutional stress would not require the actioning of a major incident plan, yet will require some communal recognition and an appropriate response. These issues often arise without warning, and can include adverse publicity about hospital practices, traumatic deaths of staff members, national disasters, a call for remembrance and memorial events, or more positively the opening of a new building.

Reflective Activity 13.1 will encourage you to critically appraise the nature of institutional stress and consider how you might respond.

Reflective Activity 13.1

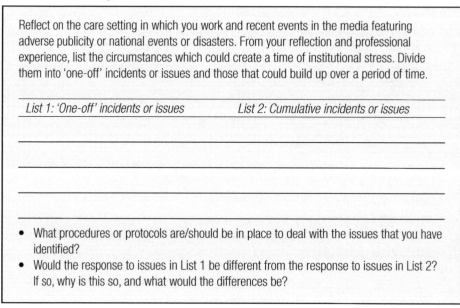

Reflect on the care setting in which you work and recent events in the media featuring adverse publicity or national events or disasters. From your reflection and professional experience, list the circumstances which could create a time of institutional stress. Divide them into 'one-off' incidents or issues and those that could build up over a period of time.

List 1: 'One-off' incidents or issues	List 2: Cumulative incidents or issues

- What procedures or protocols are/should be in place to deal with the issues that you have identified?
- Would the response to issues in List 1 be different from the response to issues in List 2? If so, why is this so, and what would the differences be?

This Reflective Activity has illustrated the fact that there are many institutional stress issues which do not fall within the remit of a 'major incident plan', but which nonetheless have to be dealt with appropriately and be in the hands of a competent individual staff member.

CHAPLAIN TO THE INSTITUTION

Through the development, professionalism, appropriate educational underpinning and recent enhancing of supervisory structures for healthcare chaplaincy, it has been clear that the role of the chaplain as a support person 'for the institution' has continued to be important. The 'institution' might be variously defined as the ward, the unit, the department, the hospice, the hospital, the primary care trust or a wider geographical area. As explored in Reflective Activity 13.1 above, there will be times when the well-being of the institution is threatened by a 'one-off' issue or the cumulative effect of a series of stresses or problems. It is often in these circumstances that the institution will turn to the chaplain, with the expectation that he or she will know what to do, will respond appropriately and will do so on behalf of the institution itself.

The UK Board of Healthcare Chaplaincy, in its *Spiritual and Religious Care Capabilities and Competences for Healthcare Chaplains*, states in Capability 3.3 that 'The chaplain is aware of his or her role in the hospital or unit's major incident plan, and responds to staff issues and events that need a communal recognition and action.'[6]

Reflective Activity 13.2 will lead you to consider what your responses and action might be.

Reflective Activity 13.2

Access and read the competences listed in the UK Board of Healthcare Chaplaincy's Capability 3.3, and then answer the following questions:
- How does your reflection on this set of competences correlate with Lists 1 and 2 which you created in Reflective Activity 13.1?
- How would you respond to the incidents or events that you listed in Reflective Activity 13.1?

The challenges of chaplaincy to the institution are many and varied. For example, the opening of a new paediatric wing, the death of the hospital's Chief Executive, a remembrance event in a neonatal unit, and a stressful period in a department or ward are just some of the challenges to which chaplains have had to respond. Services of dedication, thanksgiving and remembrance can be used creatively to the benefit of the whole institution. However, a more structured response can sometimes prove effective. Following a very public media campaign on the retention of organs from deceased children, one trust used its chaplains to answer all calls to the helpline. This proved very effective in meeting the needs of very distressed and angry relatives.[7] Chaplaincy to the institution therefore constantly calls for a creative, sincere and informed response.

INDIVIDUAL AND COLLECTIVE MORALE

The chaplain will be expected to be a resource for the provision of an ethical, theological and pastoral response to the 'mood' or circumstances of the institution, and to offer actions in response to what is around. Such a resource can only be a product of a chaplain who is fully engaged with the rise and fall of the institution's life, through regular engagement with individuals and the institution as a whole. Consequently, responses to unplanned events that have an impact on healthcare institutions will have an appropriateness which is born out of the knowledge of the nature of that institution and its people. As has been outlined above, such responses may take the form of the creation of corporate acts of spiritual significance, but in a wider context will explore and express ways in which a spiritual and religious perspective can be offered to healthcare institutions.

As has already been stated, chaplaincy services have a significant contribution to make when a major incident has been declared, and therefore policies and procedures relating to major incidents should include chaplaincy services. In addition, events in the hospital or unit, external events, world disasters and personal events can create individual or collective needs which threaten the well-being of individuals and the morale of all, to which the chaplain may be best placed to respond. It does not matter whether pastoral care is offered in a one-to-one supportive encounter, or in a suitable communal ceremony. The whole institution will benefit from every level of responsiveness to aspects of low morale.

It is important also, when major communal events are to be planned, that consideration is given to involving representatives of the different local faith communities and belief groups. This is not for reasons of political correctness, but rather because if the healthcare institution is to truly serve the whole community, the whole breadth of that community should be represented when the institution acts on its behalf.

Reflective Activity 13.3 will encourage you to think this through.

Reflective Activity 13.3

From your experience of your own clinical setting, reflect on the following:
* What would you recognise as the signs of low morale in a team?
* What might be put in place to ensure that low morale is addressed before it becomes a more acute problem?
* What might be the effective ways of addressing low morale in the short and longer term?

Engagement with a team will allow the chaplain to know what is happening, and therefore to have an idea of what might be the causes of team stress. However, perhaps more importantly, it will also allow a sensitive chaplain to be aware of changes in atmosphere and mood, which might indicate an issue that needs to be addressed. Such needs might, for example, be the personal circumstances of a member of staff (e.g. a sick relative, a marriage break-up, a financial problem), a management issue (e.g. a disciplinary matter), an enforced redundancy, poor communication of major decisions, a workload issue (e.g. a shortage of staff during a period of bad weather), illness on the ward (e.g. *Clostridium difficile*, MRSA) or a major drug error.

Opportunities for a 'critical incident review', for example, might allow a problem of low morale to be addressed and learned from, such that procedures and practices can be adjusted to ensure that such a threatening issue does not recur. The chaplain may have a positive facilitation role in these processes.

If the chaplain is to be responsive to morale issues, this has to be predicated by regular staff contact, giving insight into and corporate ownership and understanding of significant factors that affect the morale of the unit, ward, department or institution as a whole. As a result, the morale of the unit may be enhanced by raising issues and concerns with managers without breaking individual confidences, because the unit has trust in the objectivity, availability, professionalism and competence of the chaplain involved.

Moreover, through links with local communities, patients, carers and staff, chaplains can gain appropriate insight and experience that will allow them to be used legitimately as an experienced ethical resource to inform changes in healthcare service and provision. Awareness of issues or events that affect the morale or functioning of the unit which requires management engagement to resolve (e.g. managing change or communication issues) may find the chaplain acting as an appropriate resource or mediator. Requests for consultation on ethical issues relating to restructuring of services, changes in buildings, local priorities and working practices, impact on patients, carers and staff, or equality and diversity issues, would also fall appropriately within the chaplain's remit as a support for the institution and its welfare.

The unfolding case scenario and related reflective activities which follow will serve to illustrate the complexity of the chaplain's role in dealing with a multi-faceted issue, and the circumstances which change over time for the chaplain and the healthcare team.

CASE SCENARIO 13.1

Emily is a popular member of a healthcare team. As a pharmacy technician, she has involvement with and oversight of four wards. She is known, liked and respected by a wide range of healthcare professionals, and is always viewed as being efficient, personable and hard-working. No one in any of the healthcare teams knows Emily particularly well, and although she joins in activities external to the healthcare setting (such as the Christmas dance, farewell drinks, and the like), her personal circumstances are not generally known. Despite having been on the staff for 6 years, Emily hasn't revealed much of herself to anyone else, including her line manager (the senior pharmacist), preferring to keep discussions to work-related topics. She is known to have high standards, and is considered to be a 'bit of a perfectionist'. All that is known about her home circumstances is that she cycles to work, she lives with her elderly mother, and she is unattached. There have been rumours that she is gay, and although these remain unconfirmed, this has never been an issue about which there has been much anxiety. A staff 'party' has been arranged in the unit rest-room at the end of the Christmas Eve day shift, before members of the team depart for the Christmas break. Surprisingly, there is no sign of Emily. No one knows where she is, although it is confirmed that her bike is still in the rack by the main door. She is nowhere to be found. Much anxiety is expressed, as Emily hasn't turned up by the time people are planning to leave. Security is called, and a thorough search takes place. Emily is found dead in the linen store, having hanged herself with a curtain cord from the topmost slatted wooden self. It is later discovered that she had been dead for two hours. No one is sure what to do, but someone pages the chaplain.

Reflective Activity 13.4

Following Case Scenario 13.1 above, you are paged as the hospital chaplain and called to the rest-room to meet the staff who are gathered together.
- What would you anticipate the staff might be thinking and experiencing?
- What might you be expected to do?

CASE SCENARIO 13.1 CONTINUED

In the days and weeks following Emily's death the chaplain is more specifically involved in pastoral and staff support. The day after the incident she is contacted by Emily's cousin who, given the frailness of Emily's mother, has the responsibility of arranging the funeral. The chaplain is asked to visit Emily's mother and subsequently to conduct Emily's funeral. In the New Year, she receives a request from the senior pharmacist to meet and talk about what has happened. The senior pharmacist confesses to having known that Emily was depressed, although she was not privy to the reasons why, and she feels intense guilt that she 'should have seen the signs' and that she 'failed to do anything about it'.

Two months later the chaplain is contacted by a member of the nursing team, who indicates that Emily had told her shortly before she killed herself that she had 'major money worries' and commented that 'life wasn't worth living'. She was terrified that the money trouble would 'get back to her mother', but the whole situation was becoming unbearable. The nurse considered that the discussion had been confidential, but is now agonising over whether she should have done something more. 'If I'd been of more help, maybe she would still be here ...'

Some months later a new pharmacy technician is recruited, and the chaplain is asked, as part of his orientation, to give him some background about what has happened recently.

This continuing case scenario provides an example of the complex pastoral encounters that can be the norm following a significant event.

Reflective Activity 13.5 will guide you in thinking about how you might respond in each of these encounters.

Reflective Activity 13.5

Recognising the growing complexity of Case Scenario 13.1, use the following questions to consider how you would respond in each of the four pastoral encounters.
- How would you respond to the request to visit Emily's mother and conduct the funeral?
- How would you seek to support the senior pharmacist?
- How would you seek to support the nurse who is struggling with the issue of confidentiality?
- How would you approach the conversation with the new pharmacy technician, and how much information would you consider revealing?

There are many issues which might be considered here. For example, what is the relationship between Emily's cousin and her mother, and is there a possibility of the mother being excluded from any decision making? What will the nature of the funeral be (secular or religious)? Might it be a 'healing event' for Emily's colleagues? How does the senior pharmacist process her guilt, and could this be a symptom of guilt that is being experienced by others but not expressed? What are the issues of confidentiality? Would things be different if, for example, Emily's sexuality was involved or if there was a hint of criminal activity? Should the events surrounding Emily's death be solely for her former colleagues to process, or should they be explored with future staff, and what might be the balance between these two possibilities?

This unfolding case scenario illustrates the complexity of the chaplain's role in dealing with the many facets of an issue, which will affect a team differently over time, and will be dealt with by individuals in a variety of ways. It also confirms that many circumstances in which a chaplain might be involved do not lend themselves to instant solutions or a clear understanding of what the chaplain can do, but instead show the need for continued involvement and sensitivity, and a willingness to be flexible and adaptable to ever changing pictures.

CARING FOR THE CARERS, SUPPORTING THE SUPPORTERS

Although staff support cannot and should not always be in the hands of just one person, it is clear that the chaplain, as the spiritual care lead, will often be the professional who is turned to in order to 'make sense of' an issue that affects the whole institution, or simple to 'hold' the issue on behalf of the whole institution. It should be remembered, therefore, that such a person is also vulnerable, and will need both to acknowledge their own need for support, and to expect such support to come from the mutuality of the team.

When talking about cricket, Thomas Hughes wrote in *Tom Brown's Schooldays* that 'It's more than a game. It's an institution.'[8] It would be equally true to say of healthcare that 'It's more than just service delivery. It's about the institution.' And if this is true, the institution and the people within it need much care, nurture and responsiveness to their needs – hence the importance of chaplaincy to the institution.

FURTHER READING

Familiarise yourself with the policy and procedures in your hospital or unit with regard to the chaplaincy role when a major incident is declared or a significant event is recognised.

Familiarise yourself with the *NHS Emergency Planning Guidance*, which was published in July 2009, and is accessible at www.dh.gov.uk/publications, or directly from www.dh.gov.uk/prod_consum_dh/groups/dh_digitalassets/documents/digitalasset/dh_103563.pdf

Access the websites of the professional chaplaincy bodies (e.g. www.ahpcc.org.uk, www.sach.org.uk, www.healthcarechaplains.org, www.eurochaplains.org) and familiarise yourself with the available guidance on special events such as memorial services, dedications, etc.

REFERENCES

1 NHS Education for Scotland. *Spiritual Care Matters: an introductory resource for all NHS Scotland staff.* Edinburgh: NHS Education for Scotland; 2009.

2 Alfred R. *Spirituality at work.* Presented at First International Conference on Organisational Spirituality, University of Surrey, Guildford, 22–24 July 2002.

3 NHS Education for Scotland. *Spiritual Care Matters: an introductory resource for all NHS Scotland staff,* op. cit.

4 Foundation for Workplace Spirituality. www.workplacespirituality.org.uk/welcome (accessed January 2011).

5 Department of Health. *NHS Emergency Planning Guidance: interim national strategic guidance.* London: Department of Health; 2009.

6 UK Board of Healthcare Chaplaincy. *Spiritual and Religious Care Capabilities and Competences for Healthcare Chaplains.* Cambridge: UK Board of Healthcare Chaplaincy; 2009. p. 23.

7 Coutts F, Nelson J. Organ retention: Helpline experiences. *Scottish Journal of Healthcare Chaplaincy* 2004; **4:** 10–13.

8 Hughes T. *Tom Brown's Schooldays.* Oxford: Oxford University Press; 1989 edition, cited in the *Liverpool Care Pathway: standards and guidelines.* Liverpool: Marie Curie Palliative Care Institute. www.liv.ac.uk/mcpcil (accessed January 2011).

Index